THE ENCYCLOPEDIA OF Biochemic Formulas

(A Quick Remedy Finder)

- *2000 Plus Biochemic Salt Formulas*
- *Biochemic Tissue Salts Therapy*
- *Biochemic Philospohy & Healing Art*

By

Professor Dr.
Saif-ud-Din Saif
MBBS, MPH, RMP, RHMP.
Professor of Community Medicine

Cell Phone / Whatsapp: +92321-5827435
email: drsaif1919@gmail.com

COPYRIGHTS
(All rights of publication and translation of this book are reserved with the writer)

Author:
Professor Doctor
SAIF-UD-DIN SAIF
M.B;B.S, M.P.H, RMP, RHMP.

1. Graduate of Army Medical College, Rawalpindi (1982)
2. Graded Specilaist in Community Medicine (AFPGMI)
3. MPH (Master of Public Health) (UHS-Lahore)
4. Professor of Community Medicine.
5. Qualified in the fields of Allopathic and Homoeopathic systems of medicine.
6. Fields of special interest: Herabl system, Radiesthesia and Acupressure.
7. Author of many books.
8. 24 years of teaching experience at M.B;B.S. and post graduate level in various medical colleges and universities of Pakistan.

Cell Phone / Whatsapp: +92321-5827435
email address: drsaif1919@gmail.com

Other Books of Author:
1. Pharmacology: Classification and Doses *(Allopathy)*.
2. Rahnuma-e-Homeopath (Urdu).
3. Allergy-Allopathic and Homoeopathic Treatment (Urdu).
4. Research papers and articles on various topics.
5. English to Urdu and Urdu to English, Dictionary of Herbs *(under publication)*.
6. Repertory of mother tinctures *(under publication)*

Table of Contents

Preface	4
Introduction to biochemic science	4
Biochemic tissue salts, biochemic science of healing	7
List of 12 biochemic salts	8
Functions of 12 biochemic salts	9
Additional biochemic salts	10
Healing principles by Dr Sheussler	11
Introduction to tissue salts and mechanism of healing	12
Mechanism of healing	13
How tissue salts restore the health	14
How tissue salts work in the body	15
Distribution of salts in various tissues of body	17
Healthy cells, Healthy body	18
Disease	20
Importance and role of tissue salts	21
Adverse effects of deficiency of tissue salts	23
Benefits of biochemic science	24
The role of symptoms?	25
How the tissue salts are prepared	27
Administration of tissue salts to the patients	27
Finding the appropriate salt?	28
Selection of biochemic salt	29
Selection of the potency	31
How to use this book	32
Final Book - A to Z Diseases, Symptoms, Organs, Modalities, Causations with Biochemic Formulas	36

PREFACE

In the name of Allah, the most Beneficent the most Merciful

Praise be to ALLAH, the Lord of the Universe, and greetings and blessings on MUHEMMED, the Last of the Prophets, and all the Prophets as well as their household and companions.

This book provides comrehensive and most accurate information about the science and art of healing with the help of biochemic tissue salts. Tissue salts are the basic body building units and vital ingredients of human body. These salts not only make the whole body but they also play a vital role in maintaining the integrity of the body and its functions.

It has been observed that the complicated cases do not respond well or at all to the single biochemic salt, probably due to wrong selection of salt or due to the pollution of air with trace quantities of toxic substances, cigarette smoking and passive smoking. Tobacco chewing, drug ingestion, background radiation, chlorination and pollution of drinking water, adulteration of food and preservatives; other chemicals in food and beverages also antidote the effects of tissue salts. Aluminum added in diet from cooking utensils, from aluminum foils, from inner lining of packed milk and juices, is also a very hazardous metal. Above mentioned poisonous substances create a block in the process of cure. It necessitates the use of antidote tissue salts and blood purifiers (before starting the proper treatemnt) to neutralise the effects of such pollutants and barriers in the way of cure and complementary salts to augment the action of the main salt. Usage of different types of medicines by the patient in past also needs to be antidoted. In addition to that (in resistant cases) the body has to be detoxicated (at least for 3 days) before starting the tissue salts therapy. The formula, **Antidote to Poisons and Detox** (under alphabet A) is quite useful for this purpose.

It has been observed that some patients need one salt only (although most of the salts already contain two salts), but majority of the patients need more than one tissue salts, either in succession or in combination. Whether to use a single salt or a combination in a patient, depends upon the knowledge, expertise and experience of the physician. Most of the formulas has been devised and checked with the help of radionic system of therapy as well.

This book will definitely help the practitioners in curing the patients in a much better, speedy and convenient way. It will also contribute to the cause of the profession.

Formulas have following advantages as well:

1. Immediate curative and palliative response have been observed. Thus, it saves the time and satisfies the patients and the doctor.
2. Results are better and permanent.
3. No aggravation or healing crisis occurs.
4. Complicated cases respond better to a combination than a single salt. Thus, combinations have a wider and deeper spectrum of action than a single salt.
5. Most of the formulas in this book have been carefully and repeatedly tested and verified by radiesthesia.
6. In many cases tissue salts behave better in a formula than they act when applied alone.
7. No toxic side effects have been observed in the potency range specified in this work.
8. By repeated usage of formulas and with experience, one can attain the expertise to select the single salt out of a well selected formula.

9. Tissue salts can also prevent various communicable diseases, non-communicable diseases and degenerative diseases. Communicable diseases includes bacterial and viral diseases and non-communicable diseases include cancer, diabetes, and hypertension. The tissue salts for this purpose are mentioned under respective headings.

I wish to express my appreciation and gratitude to the readers of my previous books on Homoeopathy.

Suggestions from readers are most welcome for further improvement and refinement.

I present this work to the profession with a pride, confidence and hope that practitioners will use these formulas in their clinical practice and have results better than ever before, *In-sha-Allah (GOD-willing)*.

Professor DR
SAIF-UD-DIN SAIF
MBBS, MPH, RMP, RHMP.
Professor of Community Medicine.

Islamabad, Pakistan
5th July, 2024.

Email address: drsaif1919@gmail.com
Cell: +92 3215827435

BIOCHEMIC TISSUE SALTS

The human body is mainly omposed of 12 salts. These salts not only play a vital role in construction of the body tissues and organs but these are also essential for the promoting and maintain the physical, mental, spiritual health and social health.

Biochemic Science of Healing

(Twelve Tissue Remedies)

History Of The Tissue Remedies

Dr Christian Friedrich Samuel Hahnemann (1775-1843), a German physician was the first person who discovered that human body was mainly composed of twelve salts and that the deficiency of theses inorganic cell salts was the cause of various diseases.

He also discovered the healing effects of these salts for various ailments. He was the first person who mentioned about the disease causing and disease curing effects of the twelve tissue salts. He was an allopathic pysicianin who also invented the Homoeopathic science and art of healing. After Dr. Hahnemann, following doctors made contributions in develoing the biochemic science.

1. Dr Constantine Hering, father of Homeopathy in USA (1800-1880).
2. Dr Grauvogl, German allopathic physician (1811-1877).
3. Dr Lorbacher, German allopathic physician, Dr J.T O'Coner, and Dr M Docetti Walker.

Role of Dr W H Schuessler (1821-1898)

A German physician who thoroughly tested, proved and introduced this system as a comprehensive science in 1873. He was the one who laid down the healing principles of biochemic science. He named and presented the twelve principal inorganic micronutrient mineral salts.

12 Biochemic Salts

Names	Abbreviation
1. Calcarea fluoricum	Calc. fluor. (Calcium fluoride)
2. Calcarea phosphoricum	Calc.phos. (Calcium phosphate)
3. Calcarea sulphuricum	**Calcarea sulph.** (Calcium sulphate)
4. Ferrum phosphoricum	**Ferrum phos.** (Ferrum phosphate)
5. Kalium muriaticum	**Kali. mur.** (Potassium chloride)
6. Kalium phosphoricum	**Kali. phos.** (Potassium phosphate)
7. Kalium sulphuricum	**Kali. sulph.** (Potassium sulphate)
8. Magnesium Phosphoricum	**Mag. phos.** (Magnesium phosphate)
9. Natrum muriaticum	**Natrum mur.** (Sodium chloride)
10. Natrum phsophoricum	**Natrum phos.** (Sodium phosphate)
11. Natrum sulphuricum	**Natrum sulph.** (Sodium phosphate)
12. Silicea	**Silicea**

Main Functions of Tissue Salts

Calc. fluor.	Tissue Elasticity Restorer
Calc.phos.	Cell Restorer and Regeneration
Calcarea sulph.	Blood cleansing and Purifier; Anti-pus agent
Ferrum phos.	Anti-inflammatory
Kali. mur.	Detoxifying agent
Kali. phos.	Nerve and brain cells tonic
Kali. sulph.	Metabolism and Pancreas disorders
Mag. phos.	Pain of all types and Cramps
Natrum mur.	Water distributor & Fluid balance, abnormal fluid exudations from epithelium and in serous sacs
Natrum phos.	pH balance manitenance, Acidity disorders
Natrum sulph.	Liver disorders and Water eliminator
Silicea	Skin disorders Connective tissue disorders

Additional Biochemic Salts

After 12 tissue salts of Dr. Schuessler, with the advancement of science, following 21 additional tissue salts (in trace quanitities) were also discovered to be the ingredients of human body.

1. Kalium arsenicum
2. Kalium bromatum
3. Kalium iodatum
4. Lithium muriaticum
5. Magnesium sulfuricum
6. Calcarea sulfuricum
7. Cuprum arsenicosum
8. Kalium aluminum sulfuricum
9. Zincum muriaticum
10. Calcarea carbonicum
11. Natrium bicarbonicum
12. Asrenicum iodatum
13. Aurm muriaticum natronatum
14. Selenium
15. Kali bichromicum
16. Natrium vanadinicum
17. Cobaltum metallicum
18. Niccolum metallicum
19. Stannum metallicum
20. Natrium boracicum
21. Molybdenum sulfuricum

Healing Principles by Dr Scheussler

1. Our body is composed of water, organic compounds and inorganic substances or minerals. The inorganic minerals in small quantities play a vital role to activate all chemical reactions in the body and rebuilding the body by replacing continuously the waste products from the body to keep it in the state of health.
2. Disease does not occur and body remains healthy if cell metabolism is normal.
3. Cell metabolism is in turn normal if nutrients are provided to every cell in the required amounts and they work in normal way.
4. Nutritional substances are either of an organic or inorganic nature.
5. The ability of the body to absorb, assimilate, utilize the nutrients inside the cells and the process to excrete the waste materials from cells is impaired if there is a deficiency or improper functioning of the tissue salts in the body cells, blood and body organs.
6. The salts heal the body in two ways. In some cases the tissue salts make up the deficiency and let the cells function in the proper way. In other patients, the tissue salts are present in normal quantity in the body but they can not perform their function in normal way. In these cases, the salts given in potentised form correct the functioning of the already present salts in the cell.
7. Adequate cell nutrition may be restored and cell metabolism can be kept normal by continuously supplying the required (inorganic) tissue salts to the organism in a finely diluted assimilabe form.

Twelve Tissue Salts

Introduction

1. Biochemistry means the chemical reactions occurring in living organisms. It is also called as "chemistry of living tissues."
2. "Biochemical salts" are also called as "tissue salts" or "cell salts" because they are present in every cell and tissue of the body. They are also called "physiological function remedies" as their presence in optimum quantity is essential for all normal physiological functions of the body. They are twelve in number.
3. They are the constituent parts of every cell, blood and every organ of human body. They are also present in all of the food items like proteins, carbohydrates, vegetables, cereals, fruits and nuts.
4. Twelve biochemic salts work together to maintain the normal structure and function of each and every cell and organ of the body and maintain the state of physical and mental health.
5. Their deficiency in the body cells leads to underfunctioning of various systems of body, which in turn leads to various physical and mental disorders.

MECHANISM OF HEALING

1. The twelve biochemal salts directly heal the body by providing its constituent salts in potentized form and in the required quantity.
2. These salts enable the various systems of body to maintain health and promote the health, prevent the diseases and enable the immune system to be ready to fight the disease causing agents.
3. They directly correct the deficiency of salts in the body, by providing the same salts (in potentized or dyanamized form) which make, maintain, protect and heal the body.
4. They also activate the already present salts to function properly.
5. No side effects are observed, as these salts are constituent part of the body and are also present in the diet and they are given in very small or trace quantities.
6. Tissue salts can not be synthesized in the body, therefore they have to be provided from the natural sources.

HOW TISSUE SALTS RESTORE THE HEALTH

1. The normal structure and functions of all organs of the body depend upon the presence of adequate quantity and proper ratio of these tissue salts.
2. These salts are essential for maintaining the normal integrity of the structure and normal function of the body.
3. Any disturbance in body function due to deficiency or suboptimal functioning of these salts makes the body weak and vulnerable to various diseases.
4. The disease phenomenon speaks or manifests itself through various altered/abnormal feelings, emotions, sensations, symptoms and signs, which help the physician in selecting the appropriate tissue salt.
5. The disease can be prevented, rectified and health can be restored by using the same tissue salts in small quantities and in potentized form.

HOW THE CELL SALTS WORK IN THE BODY

1. The major portion of tissue salts provided by the foods is absorbed in the mouth and remaining part is absorbed in large intestine and enters the blood circulation. The salts are transported through blood circulation to each and every cell of the body. Cells keep the brain, heart, liver, endocrine and other systems healthy which in turn play the main role in distribution and balance of the salts.
2. The nutrients required for body building, energy production and normal functioning are organic and inorganic substances. These substances serve as body building blocks and also maintain the normal anatomical structure and and physiological functions of body.
3. Body cells and tissues are made and maintained by the tissue salts in the presence of oxygen, water, minerals and other nutrients.
4. Tissue salts play a vital role in metabolism. They synthesize, utilize and maintain the balance among organic substances like carbohydrates, proteins, fats, vitamins, minerals, hormones and enzymes.
5. All the destructive chemical reactions in body cells are termed as 'Catabolism' and all the constructive chemical reactions are called 'Anabolism'.
6. Sum total of all the constructive and destructive chemical reactions occurring in the body is called as 'metabolism'. It is sum total of anabolism and catabolism.

7. With the formation of new cells, the old cells keep on dying when oxidation process utilizez and destroys organic substances in the cells.
8. The combustion of organic substances produces the energy required for various body functions and also produces urea, uric acid, sulphuric acid, phosphoric acid, lactic acid, carbonic acid and water. These are the waste products.
9. Sources of waste products in body:
    a. Urea, uric acid, creatinine and sulphuric acid are chief waste products of proteins in the body.
    b. Phosphoric acid is produced by the metabolism of lecithin present in nervous tissue, brain, spinal cord and blood cells.
    c. Lactic acid is formed by metabolism of milk and milk products and it breaks down into carbonic acid and water. Lactic acid is also released from muscles and blood.
    d. These waste products are conveyed to the gall bladder, lungs, kidneys, bladder and skin for excretion via urine, faeces, respiration and skin.
    e. The waste products are transported to the excretory organs through the blood circulation and lymphatic channels.

DISTRIBUTION OF TISSUE SALTS

IN VARIOUS BODY TISSUES

Tissue salts are present all over the body but some salts are present in larger quantities in some organs than in the other organs. Examples are given below.

Brain and nerve cells	Mag. phos, Kali. phos, Natrum mur, Ferrum phos., Calc.phos.
Endocrine glands	Kali.phos, Natrum sulph, Calc.flor.
Heart	Ferrum phos, Calc.sulph, Natrum sulph, Calc.flor.
Liver	Calc.sulph, Kali.sulph, Natrum sulph, Silicea
Lungs	Mag.phos, Natrum phos, Kali.mur, Calc.flor.
Muscle cells	Mag. phos, Kali. phos, Natrum, Ferrum, Kali. mur.
Connective tissue cells	Silicea, Calc.phos.
Elastic tissue cells	Calc.fluor., Calc.phos.
Bone cells	Calc.phos, Mag.phos, Clac.fluor.
Cartilage and Mucus Cells	Natrum mur.
Natrum. mur.	All solid and fluid parts of the body.
Hair	Ferrum phos, Natrum mur, Calc.sulph, Silicea.
Crystalline Lens of eye	Natrum mur, Kali. mur, Calc.sulph, Calc. fluor.
Ovaries	Calc. phos, Ferr. phos, Kali. phos, Natrum sulph, Nat. mur, Kali. sulph, Kali. mur, Calc. flor.
Testes	Kali. phos, Nat. sulph, Nat. mur, Calc. flor, Silicea

HEALTHY CELLS-HEALTHY BODY

1. The normal cell metabolism (constructive and destructive chemical processes) of foods and water, occurs inside all the cells of various body organs.
2. The oragnaic and inorganic nutrients are supplied to the tissues so that nutrients in cells are replenished, new cells are produced and old cells die and are replaced by new ones and the waste products are excreted out of the tissues into the blood which in turn transports these to excretory oragns.
3. The food consists of carbohydrates, proteins, fats, minerals, vitamins, water and trace elements. In our body the carbohydrates are converted into glucose, the proteins into amino acids and fats into fatty acids. All the above mentioned substances are supplied to all the body cells through blood circulation. They are all utilized in the cells by chemical reactions to maintain the cell structure and function, production of heat, energy, growth, immunity and other body functions.
4. The constructive chemical reactions are called anabolism and the destructive chemical reactions are called catabolism and overall process is termed as metabolism.
5. The end products of chemical reactions in the cells are certain wastes and toxic materials like urea, uric acid, creatinine, carbon dioxide, phosphates, sulphates and water. The waste products are poisonous to the body and has to be removed from body to maintain the health.
6. If all of the above mentioned functions are occurring in a normal way and waste products are rapidly and

completely removed from the body, only then the individual can live a normal physical, mental, socially and spiritually productive life, and only then it is called as the state of health.

DISEASE

1. Health depends on normal structure and function of body cells and disease is caused by abnormal or altered function of the cells.
2. Disease process occurs when the deficiency of essential nutrients and tissue salts occurs in the diet or excessive amounts of salts are consumed due to undue physical or mental stress or wasted from stomach or any other organ. The deficiency leads to disturbance of chemical reactions occurring in the cells. Blood loss or loss of vital fluids also leads to deficiency. (Of course other factors also contribute in causation of disease).
3. As a result of disturbance in chemical reactions in cells:
   a. the process of formation of new cells does not occur,
   b. the old cells are not replaced, and
   c. waste materials produced by the cells are not removed from cells into the blood circulation, and
   d. poisonous waste products are not ultimately removed out from blood circulation and body.
4. Waste products ike bilirubin, urea, uric acid, creatinine, etc. are highly toxic and accumulation of such waste products in the body disturbs all the normal chemical functions (physiology) of the body and causes various pathological changes or diseases in different organs and may lead to organ failure if left untreated.

IMPORTANCE AND ROLE OF TISSUE SALTS

1. Biochemic salts are essential for making the new cells and maintaining their normal function. Cells are the building blocks of the body.
2. Cells make the tissues and tissues make the organs of the body. Healthy structure and function of all oragans of the body makes a healthy person.
3. In case of a disease, providing the tissue salts to the cells in proper quantity replenishes the deficiency and restores the health.
4. A proper or optimum tissue salts balance is essential for normal cell structure and function. They are also essential for maintenance of good health, protection from diseases, healing from diseases and prolonging physical and mental health, effeciency and well being.
5. Vitamims, enzymes, proteins, carbohydrates and fats can only perform their functions properly if tissue salts are also present in the body in optimum amount. Thus the tissue salts are vital and essential constituents of the body.
6. A healthy body has a healthy mind and thus leads a healthy physical, mental, spiritual, social and economically productive life.
7. The requirement of tissue salts is increased during exercise, physical or mental stress, disease, pregnancy and lactation.
8. An optimal level of tissue salts is necessary for:
    a. Maintaing and promoting the normal physical, mental and emotional health.

b. Preventing the diseases and prolonging the life.
c. Healing the body from various diseases.
d. Essential for maintaining the healthy structutre and function of the body tissues and organs.
e. Essential for digestion, absorption and assimilation of foods and water in body. Assimilation means 'the process of food and water being digested, absorbed and becoming a part of the body.'

Effects of Deficiency of Tissue Salts

1. Defienecy of tissue salts leads to various malfunctions in the cell metabolism, which in turn lead to various diseases.
2. Deficiency of one salt disturbs the functions of other salts also and the body metabolism and function as a whole as well.
3. It results into physical diseases and emotional or mental health problems.

How Deficiency of Salts Occurs

1. In addition to maintaining all the body processes, every cell performs its specific role in the specific organs.
2. Cell salts are present in normal or adequate proportions in all of the the natural foods.
3. Deficient food intake or processing, refinement, addition, fortification and adulteration of foods can disturb their natural and balanced salt proportions.
4. Chemical fertilizers and pesticide sprays also disturb the quality and quantity of the salts and other nutrients present in our foods and thus make the diet inadequate.
5. Diseases of digestive tract lead to malabsorption of salts present in diet.
6. Psychological stress, anorexia, anxiety, grief, fear and other emotional problems also lead to deficiency or disturbed function of salts.

Benefits of Biochemic Science

1. It is a natural, quite comprehensive healing medicine and not a complementary medicine.
2. Quite effective for prevention and cure of various health disorders.
3. It is safe and useful in treating the diseases of the newborn, infants, children, youth. adults and old age.
4. Quite useful for female disorders like menstrual problems, uterine diseases, ovarian diseases and hormonal problems.
5. Quite effective for treating the male sexual disorders.
6. To correct the deficiency or functioning of various natural inorganic salts in body.
7. Has no side effects or aggravation at all, except in the case of Silicea, one has to be cautious when prescribing it especially in the patients having foreign materials implanted in the body like nails and plates in bones, shunts and stents in heart, ureter, brain and pace maker in heart.
8. Can be used for people of all ages, without any side effect, i.e., newborn to the old age.
9. Of course necessary precautions should be taken after detailed study about possible side effects of cell salts before percribing the salts to the pregnant and lactating mothers.
10. Quite safe to be administered to infants directly.
11. It can also be given to an infant indirectly by giving it to the mother and through mother milk to the infant or can be given by mixing in mother milk.
12. Can also be used for boosting the immune system and as a prophaylactic against various infectious or non-infectious diseases and epidemics.

13. Quite useful for treating the nutritional deficiency disorders, neurological and mental disorders.
14. Quite effective in treating the delayed milestones of development in children.

The Role of Symptoms?

1. Symptoms and sensations are the alarm bells or danger signals of body.
2. Through symptoms, abnormal emotions and feelings, the body tells us about deficiency or excess of certain harmful chemicals in the body cells, tissues, and organs.
3. The deficiency or excess or improper metabolism of macro-nutrients, micro-nutrients, vitamins and tissue salts lead to various symptoms and causes the external and internal pathological changes.
4. The biochemic science diagnoses (finds out) the deficiency of relevant tissue salt with the help of finding out the "totality of the case" by observing the following conditions:
    a. Physical or pathological changes in body
    b. Abnormal sensations
    c. Mental changes in body
    d. Spiritual and moral disorders
    e. By finding out the modalities. Modalities are thr factors which increase and decrease the symptoms (aggravation and amelioration of symptoms).
    f. Totality also includes the personal likings and dislikings of patient regarding eating, drinking, heat or cold and other factors.

    g. The pathological changes in the body are viewed as the results of disease and not as the cause of diseases.
5. It identifies all the physical, mental and spiritual symptoms which tell us about the malfunctioning or or nature of the disease process going on in the body tissues and organs.
6. Through these symptoms our body informs the physician to select the respective deficient salt.
7. When the salts selected with the help of symptoms are given to the patient, the deficiency is corrected, the patient is cured and thus the associated disease in the body is also cured.

How the Tissue Salts are Prepared

1. The biochemic salts are prepared by the method of trituration or serial dilution at the decimal scale.
2. 1 part of the tissue salt is added in 9 parts of sugar of milk (the lactose sugar) and then triturated or thoroughly grinded. Through this process the tissue salt is diluted 10 times. This process gives us the salt in 1x strength or 1x potency.
3. 1 part of the 1x salt is again mixed in 9 parts of lactose sugar, and 2x potency is made. Through this process the tissue salt is diluted 100 times.
4. 1 part of 2x salt is mixed in 9 parts of lactose sugar and 3x potency of salt is prepared. Through this process the tissue salt is diluted 1000 times.
5. Similarly it goes up to 6x, 12x, 30x and onwards. This process can also be carried out in alcohol, to produces potencies of various strengths.
6. When salt is diluted and grinded in lactose powder it is called as "trituration" and when it is diluted by strongly shaking in alcohol, it is called as "succession."

Administration of tissue salts

1. The biochemic salts when placed in mouth are directly absorbed into the blood stream through the mucous membranes of mouth. Remaining amount of salt goes to stomach and it is absorbed by the stomach and intestines.
2. The frequency of salts is also absorbed from mouth.
3. Biochemic salts give best results when they are used after mixing in the warm water.

Finding the Appropriate Tissue Salt

1. The physician must have complete knowledge of normal body structure (anatomy) and normal body functions (physiology) and normal body chemistry (biochemistry).
2. The physician must have the knowledge about the abnormal structure and functions of body.
3. The physician must have the knowledge about the constituent tissue salts of every part and organ of a healthy body.
4. Must know about the functions of every cell salt.
5. Must know about the symptoms, signs and sensations produced by deficiency of each tissue salt.
6. Identify the deficient salt with the help of symptoms, signs, sensations, modalities and totality of the case.
7. Prescribe the appropriate tissue salt or salts (in accurate potency) to make up the deficiency and to restore the biochemical balance.
8. The biochemical balance or normal metabolism in turn corrects the healing system of the patient (cure of patient), which in turn leads to cure of the respective disease and health of the individual.

SELECTION OF BIOCHEMIC SALT

A cuartive biochemic salt is the one which is selected by keeping the symptoms of mind of the patient at top and also considering the unique symptoms and sensations, which differentiate the patient from other patients. The process of differentiation of a patient (with the help of his unique symptoms) from other patients is called the 'individualization'. Individualization is the most important step for selection of the most accurate salt for a patient.

Selection of appropriate salt in a case depends upon:
1. Knowledge about biochemic remedies. (the drug picture).
2. Knowledge about the patient. (the disease picture and the personality type).
3. Knowledge about the patient is obtained through:
    a. The age, sex, race, religion, profession, marital status, history of past illnesses and family history.
    b. History of present illness.
    c. Life style of patient: Active or sedentary.
    d. Mental symptoms.
    e. Physical symptoms and signs.
    f. Subjective feelings and emotions.
    g. Appetite: loss of or excessive appetite.
    h. Likes and dislikes of patient.
    i. Cravings and aversions of patient.
    j. Foods and drugs that agree or disagree.
    k. Eating indigestible things.
    l. Dryness of mouth.
    m. Excessive salivation from mouth.
    n. Taste disorders.
    o. Loss of smell or altered sense of smell.

p. Excessive thirst or loss of thirst.
q. Sleep diorders: Loss of sleep, sleepiness or drowsiness.
r. History of allergy.
s. Constitution of patient.
t. Reaction to heat, cold, dryness and dampness.
u. Modalities of symptoms.
v. Past history of diseases or other problems.
w. Family history of diseases or other events.
x. Causation of the symptoms.
y. Personality type and temperament.
z. Laboratory findings and other investigations.

4. Common physical symptoms of any disease are less important in selecting the curative salt, whereas the strange, unusual symptoms unique to a patient, the symptoms of mind.
5. Subjective symptoms of a patient are the most important ones for choosing the curative salt, as these symptoms represent the patient and not the disease.
6. The likes and dislikes of a patient and modalities (factors increasing and decreasing the symptoms) also play a vital role in selection of the salt.
7. The art and skill in matching the disease picture (patient picture) with the drug picture.
8. The symptomatology or disease of the patient and laboratory and other investigations.
9. Totality of the case is completed with the help of collection of all of the above mentioned information. Remember that the best salt for the patient (not the disease) can only be selected with the help of totality of the case.

SELECTION OF POTENCY

Potency of the biochemic salt is chosen on the following considerations:
1. The depth of action of remedy.
2. The acuteness or chronicity of case.
3. The susceptibility of the patient.
4. The plane of action expected of the remedy i.e, the physical or mental level.
5. Other medicines being used by the patient concurrently.
6. Habits of patient, substance abuse, like alcohol abuse, smoking, tobacco chewing, drug addiction.
7. Level of intelligence of the patient.
8. Age and sex of the patient.
9. Presence of pathological changes in the body tissues.
10. the foreign bodies implanted in the body, like pacemaker, nail and plates, stents in heart, ureter and brain.
11. Acute or chronic disease.

HOW TO USE THIS BOOK

1. This book has been arranged in an alphabetical order to enable the reader to select the most appropriate salt or formula with the help of symptoms, diseases, organs, modalities and likes/dislikes, in minimum possible time and with least effort. This arrangement has made it especially valuable for the busy practitioners.
2. A detailed table of contents is also given in the begining of the book to easily find out the relevant topic.
3. The formulas contain three salts, which is easy to be prepared and dispensed.
4. The first or uppermost salt in the formula is the specific or near-specific for most of the patients corresponding to that rubric or symptom.
5. The salts have been given in every formula according to their curative grade, in descending order. Therefore, most of the cases respond positively to the uppermost salt; whereas remaining cases are cured by the lower two salts, if used as a single remedy.
6. Mostly the potencies recommended are 3x and 6x. In some formulas 12x potency may be tried if 3x and 6x potency fails. The formulas with 3x potency are repeated three to four times a day but may be repeated after every one to two hours in acute cases.
7. From a single formula, one salt may be given in 30x potency, and second in 6x potency, and third one in 3x potency 3-4 times daily.
8. The physician can also choose the one best salt out of the formula depending upon his knowledge, experience and the totality of the patient.

9. The salts can be given mixed together or can be given in succession or one after the other.
10. Lotions, ointments, powders and creams of salts can also be used in 1x or 3x potency.
11. Concomitant symptoms and diseases have been mentioned frequently with the chief complaint of the patient. These must be consulted to complete the '*totality*' of the case.
12. For some symptoms and diseases more than one formula has been advised. A suitable formula may be chosen out of these, according to the symptom-similarity and modalities (aggravation and amelioration).
13. Under some ailments, a general formula has been given, which is suitable for majority of cases of that disorder.
14. Those desirous of using single salt may also benefit from this work; they can easiy find the single indicated salt out of the good selected group of salts under the relevant rubric.
15. The symptoms, signs, diseases, laboratory findings and names of organs have been also given in this book, with their respective formulas, to facilitate the process of consultation. In this way it is also helpful in finding the cure for newly emerging diseases.
16. The book has been arranged in alphabetic order and in repertorial fashion so that the practitioner can learn the art of repertorising the case as well.
17. The **aggravation, causation**, and **amelioration** have been presented in detailed manner. These will be of tremendous help for individualizing the case and accurate and convenient prescribing.
18. Some important instructions:

a. Biochemic salts in 30 or 200 potency can also be used as intercurrent remedy with these formulas.
b. Homeopathic medicines, nosodes and sarcodes can also be used with the biochemic salts.
c. **Nosodes** are the potentized medicinal substances, prepared from the diseased products of living organisms. **Sarcodes** are the potentized medicines prepared from the tissues or secretions of healthy organisms. The recommended potencies of nosodes and sarcodes are 200 and 1000, at weekly or fortnightly intervals; must be given in morning hours. Commonly used nosodes are Medorrhinum, Psorinum, Syphilinum, Tuberculinum and Bacillinum. Examples of sarcodes are Cholesterinum, Insulinum, Thyroidinum.

19. Where required the cross references have been made.
20. The alphabetical order of the rubrics has made the consultation quite easy.
21. The diseases of one organ or system have also been mentioned at one place under one heading. For example, all the eye symptoms and diseases have been listed below the rubric 'EYE'. Similarly, the ear, heart, kidney, liver, nose and viral diseases have been mentioned under their respective alphabets.
22. Diseases of pregnancy, climacteric and puerperium have been mentioned separately in respective groups.

23. The biochemic salts must be preferred during pregnancy and for lactating mothers. The salts should not be repeated frequently during pregnancy.
24. Salts give excellent results in the cases who are allergic to or do not respond to homoeopathic or other remedies.
25. The parctitioners must use a medical dictionary, materia medica of biochemic salts, and books on Case-taking to get maximum benefit from this book.

A

ABDOMEN

1. Abdominal diseases (General formula)
   - Nat.phos. 6x
   - Mag.phos. 6x
   - Silicea 6x
2. Aggravation of abdominal disorders by eating
   - Calc.phos. 6x
   - Kali.phos. 6x
   - Nat.phos. 6x
3. Amelioration (relief) of abdominal disorders by:
   a. Bending double
      - Mag.phos. 6x
      - Kali.phos. 6x
      - Calc.flor. 6x
   b. Eructations, belching, burping
      - Mag.phos. 6x
      - Kali.mur. 6x
      - Silicea 6x
   c. Flatus (gas), passing
      - Nat.sulph. 6x
      - Calc.phos. 6x
      - Silicea 6x
   d. Heat applied to abdomen
      - Nat.sulph. 6x
      - Kali.sulph. 6x
      - Calc.sulph. 6x
   e. Rubbing the abdomen
      - Mag.phos. 6x
      - Natrum sulph. 6x
      - Calc.flor. 6x
4. Distended abdomen, due to gas
   - Silicea 6x
   - Calc.sulph. 6x
   - Kali.sulph. 6x

5. Cannot bear tight clothing, around abdomen
   - Nat.sulph.   6x
   - Calc.sulph.   6x
   - Silicea   6x

6. Cramps in abdomen
   - Natrum sulph.   6x
   - Kali.sulph.   6x
   - Silicea   6x

7. Distention or fullness of abdomen
   - Nat.mur.   6x
   - Kali.sulph.   6x
   - Mag.phos.   6x

8. Dropsy (abnormal fluid in abdomen) *(See Ascites)*

9. Enlarged abdomen
   a. *Adults and children*
   - Calc.sulph.   6x
   - Calc.flor.   6x
   - Silicea   6x

   b. *After delivery*
   - Kali.sulph.   6x
   - Calc.sulph.   6x
   - Silicea   6x

10. Gas in abdomen, bloatedness (Flatulence)
    - Nat.sulph.   6x
    - Nat.phos.   6x
    - Calc.sulph.   6x

11. Hardness of abdomen
    - Kali.sulph.   6x
    - Calc.sulph.   6x
    - Silicea   6x

12. Large abdomen
    a. *Due to fat deposits (obesity)*
Nat. sulph.	6x
Kali.sulph.	6x
Calc.sulph.	6x
    b. *Large abdomen, after labor*
Kali.sulph.	6x
Calc.sulph.	6x
Silicea	6x

13. Pain in abdomen
    a. *General formula*
Ferrum phos	6x
Natrum sulph.	6x
Calc.sulph.	6x
    b. *Pain in abdomen-due to Constipation*
Natrum sulph.	6x
Kali.sulph.	6x
Calc.sulph.	6x
    c. *Pain in abdomen-Cramps, griping*
Kali.phos.	6x
Mag.phos.	6x
Nat.phos.	6x
    d. *Pain in abdomen-from Flatulence (gas)*
Natrum sulph.	6x
Kali.sulph.	6x
Calc.sulph.	6x
    e. *Pain in abdomen-from Worms*
Kali.phos.	6x
Natrum sulph.	6x
Silicea	6x

14. Sensation, as if stone in abdomen
Nat.mur.	6x
Kali.mur.	6x
Calc.sulph.	6x

15. Sunken abdomen
                      Ferr.phos.   6x
                      Natrum mur.   6x
                      Kali sulph.   6x
16. Swollen, distended, abdomen
                      Nat.mur.   6x
                      Kali.mur.   6x
                      Calc.flor.   6x
17. Tenesmus and tympanitic abdomen
                      Nat.sulph.   6x
                      Kali.sulph.   6x
                      Calc.sulph.   6x
(For other abdominal disorders see gall-bladder, duodenum, intestine, liver, pancreas, spleen, stomach and ulcer).

18. Right-sided abdominal problems
                      Natrum sulph. 6x
                      Kali.sulph.   6x
                      Calc.sulph.   6x
19. Left-sided abdominal problems
                      Kali.sulph.   6x
                      Calc.sulph.   6x
                      Silicea   6x

ABORTION

1. From debility, anemia, malnutrition
                      Natrum mur.   6x
                      Kali.sulph.   6x
                      Calc.sulph.   6x
2. To prevent the tendency to abortion
                      Nat.mur.   6x
                      Kali.sulph.   6x
                      Calc.sulph.   6x
Dose: 3 times daily for 3 months before pregnancy.

3. From 2nd to 3rd month
- Kali.sulph. 6x
- Calc.sulph. 6x
- Silicea 6x

Dose: 3 times daily for 3 months before pregnancy and one dose daily during the pregnancy.

4. Due to injury or over-exertion
- Natrum mur. 6x
- Kali.sulph. 6x
- Calc.sulph. 6x

Dose: Reapeat every half hour, till the pain stops. After that 2-3 times daily, for one month.

5. Habitual abortion or from weakness
- Kali.phos. 6x
- Mag.phos. 6x
- Nat.phos. 6x

Dose: 3 times daily for 3 months before pregnancy and once daily durig pregnancy.

6. After-effects of abortion, weakness and debility
- Ferr. Phos. 6x
- Kali. phos. 6x
- Nat. mur. 6x

7. Emergency treatment to stop the abortion
- Kali.phos. 6x
- Natrum mur. 6x
- Calc.sulph. 6x

Dose: Give one dose after every hour; total 6 doses. On improvement give 3 hourly dose and on further improvement give four times daily for one month.

ABRUPT BEHAVIOR, UNPREDICTABLE

- *Kali. Phos.* 6x
- *Nat. mur.* 6x
- *Kali. mur.* 6x

ABSCESS

1. All types of abscess   Calc.sulph.   6x
       Silicea   6x
       Calc.flor.   6x

2. The following formula is to be administered in low potency (3x or 6x) if the process of suppuration is to be promoted and the pus has to be drained; and in high potency (30x) if the suppuration has to be stopped.
       Kali.sulph.   3x
       Calc.sulph.   3x
       Silicea   3x

3. Abscess, furuncle, carbuncle (before the pus is formed)
       Kali. mur.   6x
       Kali. sulph.   6x
       Calc.sulph.   6x

   (Kali.mur., Calc.sulph or Silicea 3x can also be used for external dressing mixed in vaseline).

4. If the above formula fails to abort the suppuration and pus appears, then use:
       Silicea   6x
       Calc.sulph.   6x
       Kali.sulph.   6x

5. Alveolar abscess (abscess of bony socket of tooth)
       Nat.sulph.   6x
       Kali.mur.   6x
       Calc.sulph.   6x
       (See Gums below and Gums also)

6. Anus-painful abscess
       Kali.sulph.   6x
       Nat.sulph.   6x
       Calc.sulph.   6x

7. Bones abscess (Osteomyelitis)
       Calc.flor.   6x
       Calc.phos.   6x
       Silicea   6x

8. Breast abscess (See Breasts)

9. Burrowing abscess (Hole or burrow like)
   - Kali.sulph. 6x
   - Kali. mur. 6x
   - Calc.sulph. 6x

10. Chronic abscess
    - Nat. mur. 6x
    - Kali. mur. 6x
    - Calc.sulph. 6x

11. Cystic acne-abscess, boil
    - Ferrum phos. 6x
    - Natrum sulph. 6x
    - Calc.sulph. 6x

12. Injection abscess (Abscess at the site of injection)
    - Kali.phos. 6x
    - Kali.sulph. 6x
    - Calc.sulph. 6x

13. Felon, whitlow and gathered breasts
    - Nat.sulph. 6x
    - Kali.sulph. 6x
    - Calc.sulph. 6x

14. Fistulous abscess (Fistula)
    - Kali. mur. 6x
    - Kali.sulph. 6x
    - Calc.sulph. 6x

15. Glands (lymh nodes), abscess
    - Kali. mur. 6x
    - Kali.sulph. 6x
    - Calc.sulph. 6x

16. Gums: Inflammation, gingivitis, gumboil
    - Calc.sulph. 6x
    - Nat.mur. 6x
    - Kali.sulph. 6x

17. Inflammation (Redness, swelling and pain)
    - Silicea 6x
    - Kali.sulph. 6x
    - Calc.sulph. 6x

18. Lung abscess
        Natrum sulph. 6x
        Kali sulph. 6x
        Calc.sulph. 6x
19. Peri-anal abscess (Ano-rectal abscess) *(See Anus)*
20. Periosteum (Membrane covering the bones), abscess
        Calc.sulph. 6x
        Kali. sulph. 6x
        Silicea 6x
21. Pilonidal cyst/sinus (See Pilonidal)
22. Recurrent abscess, tendency of abscess formtion
        Calc.sulph. 6x
        Kali.sulph. 6x
        Natrum sulph. 6x
23. Psoas abscess
        Calc.sulph. 6x
        Kali.sulph. 6x
        Natrum sulph. 6x
24. Stitch abscess (Abscess at the site of a stitch)
        Natrum sulph. 6x
        Kali.sulph. 6x
        Calc.sulph. 6x
25. To prevent or shorten pus formation
        Calc.sulph. 6x
        Calc.fluor. 6x
        Silicea 6x
26. Tonsils-abscess, inflammation
        Calc.sulph. 6x
        Kali.mur. 6x
        Kali. sulph. 6x
27. Pelvic abscess
        Kali. mur. 6x
        Kali. sulph. 6x
        Calc.sulph. 6x
28. Retro-pharyngeal abscess
        Kali. sulph. 6x
        Calc.sulph. 6x
        Nat.sulph. 6x

29. Scalp abscess

      Calc.sulph. 6x
      Kali. mur. 6x
      Kali. sulph. 6x

30. Weakness, extreme-with abscess

      Kali.phos. 6x
      Kali.mur. 6x
      Calc.sulph. 6x

ABSENT-MINDED, WEAK MEMORY

      Kali. phos. 6x
      Nat. phos. 6x
      Nat. sulph. 6x

ABSORBED, Buried in thoughts

      Kali. phos. 6x
      Nat. sulph. 6x
      Kali. sulph. 6x

ABSORBED, as to what would become of him

      Kali.phos. 6x
      Nat. sulph. 6x
      Calc.sulph. 6x

ABSTRACTION OF MIND

      Calc. phos. 6x
      Kali. phos. 6x
      Nat. mur. 6x

ABUSES, INSULTS OTHERS

      Kali.sulph. 6x
      Natrum Mur. 6x
      Calc.sulph. 6x

ABUSED BY OTHERs-ill effects

      Natrum mur. 6x
      Calc.sulph. 6x
      Silicea 6x

ABUSIVE LANGUAGE
Kali. mur. 6x
Nat. mur. 6x
Calc.sulph. 6x

ACIDITY (Heartburn, excess of acid in stomach)
Kali.phos. 6x
Natrum sulph. 6x
Silicea 6x

ACID REFLUX-Gastroesophageal reflux disease (GERD)
Natrum mur. 6x
Calc.sulph. 6x
Calc.flor. 6x

ACNE VULGARIS
1. All types of acne
Calc.phos. 6x
Kali.phos. 6x
Natrum mur. 6x

2. Back of the body, on
Calc.phos. 6x
Calc.sulph. 6x
Nat. mur. 6x

3. Acne-boys and girls
Nat.mur. 6x
Kali.sulph. 6x
Calc.sulph. 6x

4. Acne simplex, with or without pimples
Calc.phos. 6x
Natrum mur. 6x
Calc.sulph. 6x

5. Acne-with fast foods, fatty foods, chocolate, coffee, etc.
Kali.mur. 6x
Kali.sulph. 6x
Calc.sulph. 6x

6. Acne-with emotional problems

Kali.phos.	6x
Natrum mur.	6x
Calc.sulph.	6x

7. Acne-with gastric derangements

Natrum mur.	6x
Kali.sulph.	6x
Calc.sulph.	6x

8. Acne - with hormonal imbalance in females

Calc.sulph.	6x
Calc.flor.	6x
Silicea	6x

9. Acne-with mestrual irregularities

Ferrum phos	6x
Natrum mur.	6x
Kali sulph.	6x

10. Acne-with oily skin

Natrum mur.	6x
Natrum sulph.	6x
Kali.mur.	6x

11. Acne-with polycystic ovarian syndrome

Kali.mur.	6x
Kali.sulph.	6x
Calc.sulph.	6x

ACNE ROSACEA

Kali.phos.	6x
Natrum mur.	6x
Calc.sulph.	6x

ACQUIRED IMMUNE DEFICIENCY SYNDROME (AIDS)

Natrum sulph.	6x
Kali.sulph.	6x
Calc.sulph.	6x

ACROMEGALY

Natrum sulph.	6x
Kali.sulph.	6x
Calc.sulph.	6x

ACTINOMYCOSIS (Multiple abscesses or infection due to gram positive bacteria).

Calc.phos.	6x
Natrum mur.	6x
Kali.mur.	6x

ACUTE HAEMORRHAGIC CONJUNCTIVITIS

Natrum sulph.	6x
Kali.sulph.	6x
Calc.sulph.	6x

ACUTE LIVER FAILURE (See Liver also)

Ferrum phos.	6x
Natrum sulph.	6x
Calc.sulph.	6x

ACUTE RESPIRATORY DISTRESS SYNDROME (ARDS)

Natrum mur.	6x
Kali.sulph.	6x
Calc.sulph.	6x

Dose: in case of an emergency, give 5 doses at half hourly intervals and on improvement give 3-4 times a day.

ADHD (See Attention deficit hyperactivity disorder)
ADDICTION-(Substance abuse)
Cannabis indica (hemp, hash, marijuana) smoking
1. General formula

Kali.sulph.	6x
Calc.sulph.	6x
Silicea	6x

2. Cocaine sniffing or smoking

Kali.phos.	6x
Kali.mur.	6x
Calc.sulph.	6x

3. Ice, crystal

Kali.phos.	6x
Natrum sulph.	6x
Calc.sulph.	6x

4. Heroin smoking habit

Kali.sulph.	6x
Calc.sulph.	6x
Silicea	6x

5. Morphine eating habit

Kali.mur.	6x
Kali.sulph.	6x
Calc.sulph.	6x

6. Tobacco, chewing

Kali.sulph.	6x
Calc.sulph.	6x
Silicea	6x

7. Tobacco smoking

Kali.mur.	6x
Calc.sulph.	6x
Silicea	6x

ADDISON'S DISEASE

Calc.phos.	6x
Nat.sulph.	6x

ADENITIS *(Lymph node inflammation)*

1. General formula

Kali.mur.	6x
Calc.sulph.	6x
Silicea	6x

2. Acute adenitis

Kali.mur.	6x
Kali.sulph.	6x
Calc.sulph.	6x

3. Chronic adenitis

Kali.sulph.	6x
Calc.sulph.	6x
Silicea	6x

ADENITIS (Inflammation of lymph nodes)

LOCATION

1. Axillary lymph nodes
   - Natrum sulph. 6x
   - Kali.sulph. 6x
   - Calc.sulph. 6x
2. Cervical (neck), lymph nodes
   - Kali.sulph. 6x
   - Calc.sulph. 6x
   - Silicea 6x
3. Hilar lymph nodes in chest
   - Natrum mur. 6x
   - Natrum sulph. 6x
   - Kali.mur. 6x
4. Inguinal (groin) lymph nodes
   - Natrum mur. 6x
   - Natrum sulph. 6x
   - Kali.mur. 6x

ADENOID GLANDS - HYPERTROPHY
- Calc.flor. 6x
- Calc.phos. 6x
- Kali.mur. 6x

ADHESIONS OF INTERNAL TISSUES, with each other

(Tissues can adhere to each other with or without operations, especially in abdomen or pelvis organs)

1. General formula
   - Kali.sulph. 6x
   - Calc.sulph. 6x
   - Calc.flor. 6x
2. After operation-adhesions of visceral tissues
   - Kali.sulph. 6x
   - Calc.sulph. 6x
   - Calc.flor. 6x

3. Pleuritic adhesion
    Natrum sulph. 6x
    Kali.mur. 6x
    Kali.sulph. 6x
    Calc.sulph. 6x

ADYNAMIA-COLLAPSE (See Collapse and Weakness)

AFFECTIONATE-Diseases of sympathetic persons
    Kali.phos. 6x
    Natrum sulph. 6x
    Kali.sulph. 6x

AFTER-EFFECTS (ill-effects) of
1. Acute, exhausting diseases (Bacterial or viral)
    Kali.phos. 6x
    Natrum mur. 6x
    Silicea 6x

2. Alcohol
    Kali. Phos. 6x
    Nat. Sulph. 6x
    Calc.sulph. 6x

3. Anger
    Natrum mur. 6x
    Kali.mur. 6x
    Calc.sulph. 6x

4. Bites, of insects
    Nat.mur. 6x
    Kali.mur. 6x
    Calc.flor. 6x

5. Blows, accidents
    Kali.phos. 6x
    Calc.sulph. 6x
    Silicea 6x

6. Concussion, of head
    Kali.phos. 6x
    Natrum sulph. 6x
    Calc.sulph. 6x

7. Diabtes mellitus
        Kali.phos. 6x
        Natrum sulph. 6x
        Calc.sulph. 6x
8. Diarrhoea, dysentery, dehydration
        Kali.phos. 6x
        Natrum mur. 6x
        Calc.sulph. 6x
8. Disapponitment, from failure in examination, etc.
        Kali.phos. 6x
        Calc.sulph. 6x
        Silicea 6x
9. Disappointed love
        Natrum mur. 6x
        Calc.sulph. 6x
        Silicea 6x
10. Drugs, ill-effects
        Calc.phos. 6x
        Calc.sulph. 6x
        Silicea 6x
11. Fever, illness - ill-effects
        Kali.sulph. 6x
        Calc.sulph. 6x
        Silicea 6x
12. Fright, fear
        Calc.sulph. 6x
        Calc.flor. 6x
        Silicea 6x
13. Grief
        Kali.phos. 6x
        Calc.sulph. 6x
        Silicea 6x
14. Hepatitis A
        Natrum sulph. 6x
        Kali.sulph. 6x
        Calc.sulph. 6x

15. Hepatitis B
    Natrum sulph. 6x
    Kali.sulph. 6x
    Calc.sulph. 6x

16. Hepatitis C
    Kali.sulph. 6x
    Calc.sulph. 6x
    Silicea 6x

17. Hypertension
    Natrum mur. 6x
    Kali.mur. 6x
    Calc.flor. 6x

18. Influenza, Flu, Infectious diseases
    Kali.sulph. 6x
    Calc.sulph. 6x
    Silicea 6x

19. Insult, emotional injury, mental shock
    Kali.phos 3x
    Calc.flor. 6x
    Silicea 6x

20. Injury, trauma-physical
    Kali.sulph. 6x
    Calc.flor. 6x
    Silicea 6x

21. Jaundice, hepatitis
    Nat.sulph. 6x
    Kali.sulph. 6x
    Calc.sulph. 6x

22. Sun heat, sun-stroke
    Natrum sulph. 6x
    Kali.mur. 6x
    Calc.sulph. 6x

23. Tuberculosis
    Kali.phos. 6x
    Kali.sulph. 6x
    Calc.sulph. 6x

24. Typhoid fever
Kali.sulph.	6x
Calc.sulph.	6x
Silicea	6x

25. Vaccination or any injection
Kali.sulph.	6x
Calc.sulph.	6x
Silicea	6x

26. Vexation, worry
Kali.phos.	6x
Natrum sulph.	6x
Calc.sulph.	6x

27. Viral or bacterial diseases
Kali.sulph.	6x
Calc.sulph.	6x
Silicea	6x

AFTER-PAINS (Pains after labor)
Kali.phos.	6x
Natrum sulph.	6x
Kali sulph.	6x

AGALACTIA (Absence of mother's milk)
Calc.phos.	6x
Kali.phos.	6x
Calc.sulph.	6x

AGGRAVATION AND CAUSATION (aggravate or cause)

1. Air, cold, dry
Natrum sulph.	6x
Kali.sulph.	6x
Silicea	6x

2. Bending forward
Natrum sulph.	6x
Kali.sulph.	6x
Calc.sulph.	6x

3. Coitus, excessive sex

Ferrum phos	6x
Kali.phos.	6x
Natrum sulph.	6x

4. Damp, living houses

Natrum sulph.	6x
Kali.sulph.	6x
Calc.sulph.	6x

5. Fats

Natrum sulph.	6x
Calc.sulph.	6x
Silicea	6x

6. Fish

Natrum sulph.	6x
Kali.sulph.	6x
Calc.sulph.	6x

7. Grief

Kali.phos.	6x
Natrum sulph.	6x
Calc.sulph.	6x

8. Light

Kali.phos.	6x
Natrum sulph.	6x
Calc.sulph.	6x

9. Localised Symtoms

Kali.phos.	6x
Natrum sulph.	6x
Calc.sulph.	6x

10. Lying down

Natrum sulph.	6x
Kali.sulph.	6x
Calc.sulph.	6x

11. Lying on left side		
	Natrum sulph.	6x
	Kali.sulph.	6x
	Calc.sulph.	6x
12. Lying on right side		
	Kali.sulph.	6x
	Calc.sulph.	6x
	Silicea	6x
13. Mental exertion		
	Kali.phos.	6x
	Natrum mur.	6x
	Calc.sulph.	6x
14. Milk		
	Natrum sulph.	6x
	Kali.sulph.	6x
	Calc.sulph.	6x
15. Misdeed of others, insult		
	Kali.phos.	6x
	Natrum mur.	6x
	Calc.sulph.	6x
16. Mortification from an offence		
	Kali.phos.	6x
	Natrum sulph.	6x
	Calc.sulph.	6x
17. Morning		
	Kali.mur.	6x
	Kali.sulph.	6x
	Calc.sulph.	6x
18. Motion		
	Mag.phos.	6x
	Nat.phos.	6x
	Natrum sulph.	6x
19. Motion, continuous		
	Kali.phos.	6x
	Natrum sulph.	6x
	Calc.sulph.	6x

20. Narcotics, hash, morphine, ice, etc
　　　　　　　　　　Kali.phos.　　6x
　　　　　　　　　　Natrum mur.　6x
　　　　　　　　　　Kali.mur.　　　6x
　　　　　　　　　　Silicea　　　　6x
21. Night
　　　　　　　　　　Kali.phos.　　6x
　　　　　　　　　　Natrum sulph.　6x
　　　　　　　　　　Calc.sulph.　　6x
22. Noise
　　　　　　　　　　Kali.phos.　　6x
　　　　　　　　　　Natrum sulph.　6x
　　　　　　　　　　Calc.sulph.　　6x
23. One half of body
　　　　　　　　　　Calc.phos.　　6x
　　　　　　　　　　Kali.phos.　　6x
　　　　　　　　　　Natrum sulph.　6x
24. Open air aggravates and inside room, ameliorates
　　　　　　　　　　Kali.phos.　　6x
　　　　　　　　　　Natrum mur.　6x
　　　　　　　　　　Calc.sulph.　　6x
(Open air ameliorates, while inside room aggravates)
　　　　　　　　　　Natrum sulph.　6x
　　　　　　　　　　Kali.mur.　　　6x
　　　　　　　　　　Calc.sulph.　　6x
25. Pastry or other bakery products
　　　　　　　　　　Natrum sulph.　6x
　　　　　　　　　　Kali.sulph.　　6x
　　　　　　　　　　Calc.sulph.　　6x
26. Periodical aggravation
　　　　　　　　　　Calc.phos.　　6x
　　　　　　　　　　Kali.phos.　　6x
　　　　　　　　　　Natrum sulph.　6x
27. Rain or rainy season
　　　　　　　　　　Natrum sulph.　6x
　　　　　　　　　　Kali.sulph.　　6x
　　　　　　　　　　Silicea　　　　6x

28. Rest aggravates
	Kali.phos.	6x
	Natrum sulph.	6x
	Kali sulph.	6x

29. Riding
	Kali.phos.	6x
	Natrum sulph.	6x
	Calc.sulph.	6x

30. Right side
	Kali.phos.	6x
	Natrum sulph.	6x
	Calc.sulph.	6x

31. Rising from seat
	Kali.phos.	6x
	Mag.phos.	6x
	Calc.sulph.	6x

32. Rising
	Natrum sulph.	6x
	Kali.sulph.	6x
	Calc.sulph.	6x

33. Room aggravates, open air ameliorates
	Natrum sulph.	6x
	Kali.mur.	6x
	Calc.sulph.	6x

34. Room, heated, aggravates
	Natrum sulph.	6x
	Kali.sulph.	6x
	Calc.sulph.	6x

35. Room full of people, aggravates
	Kali.phos.	6x
	Kali.sulph.	6x
	Calc.sulph.	6x

36. Running
	Kali.phos.	6x
	Natrum sulph.	6x
	Calc.sulph.	6x

37. Sea bathing

	Kali.phos.	6x
	Natrum mur.	6x
	Calc.sulph.	6x

38. Sea side

	Natrum mur.	6x
	Calc.sulph.	6x
	Calc.flor.	6x

39. Sedentary habits

	Natrum sulph.	6x
	Kali.sulph.	6x
	Calc.flor.	6x

40. Sexual excess or coitus (both sexes)

	Kali.phos.	6x
	Natrum sulph.	6x
	Calc.sulph.	6x

41. Sitting

	Natrum sulph.	6x
	Kali.sulph.	6x
	Calc.sulph.	6x
	Silicea	6x

42. Sitting, erect

	Kali.phos.	6x
	Kali.sulph.	6x
	Calc.sulph.	6x

43. Slight causes

	Kali.phos.	6x
	Natrum sulph.	6x
	Calc.sulph.	6x

44. Smoking, tobacco chewing, gutka eating, naswaar

	Kali.phos.	6x
	Calc.sulph.	6x
	Natrum sulph.	6x

45. Sneezing

Kali.phos.	6x
Natrum sulph.	6x
Calc.sulph.	6x

46. Speaking

Kali.phos.	6x
Natrum sulph.	6x
Calc.sulph.	6x

47. Spring season

Natrum sulph.	6x
Kali.sulph.	6x
Calc.sulph.	6x

48. Standing

Kali.phos.	6x
Natrum sulph.	6x
Calc.sulph.	6x

49. Straining, overlifting, stretching

Kali.phos.	6x
Calc.sulph.	6x
Natrum sulph.	6x

50. Sun heat

Calc.phos.	6x
Kali.phos.	6x
Natrum sulph.	6x

51. Sweets, sugar

Natrum sulph.	6x
Kali.sulph.	6x
Calc.flor.	6x

52. Talking

Kali.phos.	6x
Natrum sulph.	6x
Calc.sulph.	6x

53. Thunderstorm
Kali.phos.	6x
Natrum sulph.	6x
Calc.sulph.	6x

54. Tobacco chewing
Natrum sulph.	6x
Calc.sulph.	6x
Silicea	6x

55. Tobacco Smoking and passive smoking
Kali.phos.	6x
Natrum sulph.	6x
Kali sulph.	6x

56. Touch
Kali.phos.	6x
Calc.sulph.	6x
Silicea	6x

57. Vital drains
Calc.phos.	6x
Kali.phos.	6x
Natrum sulph.	6x

58. Voice, using (speakers, singers, teachers)
Kali.phos.	6x
Natrum sulph.	6x
Calc.flor.	6x

59. Warmth, heat
Kali.phos.	6x
Natrum sulph.	6x
Calc.sulph.	6x

60. Warmth of bed
Kali.phos.	6x
Natrum sulph.	6x
Calc.sulph.	6x

61. Washing and working in water
Natrum sulph.	6x
Kali.sulph.	6x
Calc.sulph.	6x

62. Water, drinking, aggravates
         Natrum sulph. 6x
         Calc.sulph. 6x
         Kali sulph. 6x

63. Weather, cold
         Kali.sulph. 6x
         Calc.sulph. 6x
         Silicea 6x

64. Weather, hot
         Kali.phos. 6x
         Natrum sulph. 6x
         Calc.sulph. 6x

65. Wetting feet
         Kali.phos. 6x
         Natrum sulph. 6x
         Calc.sulph. 6x

AGONY, RESTLESS, TOSSING ABOUT
         Kali.phos. 6x
         Natrum mur. 6x
         Kali.sulph. 6x

AIR CASTLES, theorizing
         Kali.phos. 6x
         Natrum sulph. 6x
         Calc.sulph. 6x

AIR TRAVEL SICKNESS
         Natrum mur. 6x
         Kali.mur. 6x
         Calc.sulph. 6x

ALBUMINURIA
1. General formula
         Kali.phos. 6x
         Nat.mur. 6x
         Kali.mur. 6x

2. Pregnancy, during *(Dose: once daily)*

Nat.mur.	3x
Calc.phos.	3x
Kali.mur.	3x

ALCOHOLIC CARDIOMYOPATHY

Natrum sulph.	6x
Calc.sulph.	6x
Silicea	6x

ALCOHOLISM
1. To quit the habit

Calc.phos.	6x
Kali.phos.	6x
Natrum mur.	6x

2. To treat the ill-effects of alcohol

Kali.phos.	6x
Nat.phos.	6x
Natrum sulph.	6x

3. Delirium tremens (Confusion after withdrawal of alcohol)

Nat.mur.	6x
Kali.phos.	6x
Natrum sulph.	6x

(See Delirium as well)

ALLERGIC CONJUNCTIVITIS   See Allergies
ALLERGIC CONTACT DERMATITIS See Allergies
ALLERGIC RHINITIS   See Allergies

ALLERGIES
1. General remedy for all types of allergy

Kali.phos.	6x
Natrum mur.	6x
Kali.mur.	6x

2. Air allergy (Allergy of skin, when air strikes the skin)

Natrum sulph.	6x
Kali.sulph.	6x
Calc.sulph.	6x

3. Allergic asthma (Hay fever)

Kali.phos.	6x
Natrum mur.	6x
Kali.sulph.	6x
Calc.sulph.	6x

4. Allergy, even from anti-allergic drugs

Natrum mur.	6x
Kali.mur.	6x
Calc.sulph.	6x

5. Antibiotibiotics and other medicines

Calc.sulph.	6x
Natrum mur.	6x
Nat.sulph.	6x
Kali.mur.	6x

6. Beef allergy

Natrum mur.	6x
Kali sulph.	6x
Calc.sulph.	6x

7. Chocolate allergy

Nat. sulph.	6x
Calc.sulph.	6x
Calc. fluor.	6x

8. Cold allergy

Natrum mur.	6x
Kali.sulph.	6x
Silicea	6x

9. Contact dermatitis or atopy, allergic

Natrum mur.	6x
Kali.sulph.	6x
Calc.sulph.	6x

10. Condiments (spices) allergy

Natrum sulph.	6x
Kali sulph.	6x
Calc.sulph.	6x

11. Cosmatics, chemicals, hair dyes, soap
       Nat.mur. 6x
       Kali.sulph. 6x
       Kali.mur. 6x
12. Egg allergy
       Ferrum phos 6x
       Natrum mur. 6x
       Kali.sulph. 6x
13. Eyes, allergic conjunctivitis (redness, itching, watering)
       Natrum mur. 6x
       Kali.mur. 6x
       Calc.sulph. 6x
14. Feathers, dust, allergy or effects of
       Natrum mur. 6x
       Kali.mur. 6x
       Calc.sulph. 6x
15. Feathers, of bed, or pillow aggravate
       Natrum mur. 6x
       Kali.mur. 6x
       Calc.sulph. 6x
16. Fish-allergy
       Kali.phos. 6x
       Natrum mur. 6x
       Kali.mur. 6x
17. Food allergy
       Natrum sulph. 6x
       Kali sulph. 6x
       Calc.sulph. 6x
18. Glutin (wheat or wheat products) allergy
       Calc.phos. 6x
       Natrum mur. 6x
       Kali.mur. 6x
19. Heat allergy
       Natrum sulph. 6x
       Kali.mur. 6x
       Kali sulph. 6x

20. Honey-allergy

Calc.phos.	6x
Natrum sulph.	6x
Calc.sulph.	6x

21. Humidity, dampness or rain

Natrum mur.	6x
Nat.sulph.	6x
Kali sulph.	6x

22. Meats

Calc.phos.	6x
Nat.mur.	6x
Kali.mur.	6x

23. Metals-allergy
   a. Aluminium jewellary

Natrum mur.	6x
Calc.flor.	6x
Silicea	6x

   b. Gold allergy

Calc.sulph.	6x
Kali.mur.	6x
Natrum mur.	6x

   c. Siver allergy

Kali.sulph.	6x
Natrum sulph.	6x
Silicea	6x

24. Milk allergy

Natrum mur.	6x
Kali.mur.	6x
Calc.sulph.	6x

24. Mutton allergy

Natrum mur.	6x
Kali.mur.	6x
Kali sulph.	6x

25. Nasal allergy (Allergic rhinitis)

Natrum mur.	6x
Kali.mur.	6x
Calc.sulph.	6x

26. Onion allergy

Kali.mur.	6x
Kali.sulph.	6x
Calc.sulph.	6x

27. Potato allergy

Natrum mur.	6x
Kali.sulph.	6x
Calc.sulph.	6x

28. Poultry allergy

Natrum mur.	6x
Natrum sulph.	6x
Kali.mur.	6x

29. Respiratory allergy (sneezing, cough, breathless, catarrh)

a. *asthma (allergic)*

Nat.mur.	6x
Natrum sulph.	6x
Kali.sulph.	6x

b. *at every change of season*

Natrum mur.	6x
Natrum sulph.	6x
Kali.mur.	6x

c. *dust allergy*

Natrum mur.	6x
Kali.mur.	6x
Calc.sulph.	6x

d. *recurrent chest infections*

Calc.phos.	6x
Natrum sulph.	6x
Calc.sulph.	6x

e. *nasal allergy, cold and flu*

Kali.mur.	6x
Kali.sulph.	6x
Calc.sulph.	6x

f. *pollen (Spring season allergy)*

Natrum mur.	6x
Natrum sulph.	6x
Kali sulph.	6x

g. *sinus allergy (allergic sinusitis)*

Natrum sulph.	6x
Kali.sulph.	6x
Calc.sulph.	6x

h. *sneezing*

Natrum mur.	6x
Kali.mur.	6x
Calc.sulph.	6x

i. *throat allergy, recurrent infection*

Natrum sulph.	6x
Kali.sulph.	6x
Calc.sulph.	6x

30. Skin allergy

a. *General formula*

Natrum sulph.	6x
Kali.sulph.	6x
Calc.sulph.	6x

b. *Air allergy (allergy when air strikes the skin)*

Natrum sulph.	6x
Kali.sulph.	6x
Calc.sulph.	6x

c. *Allergic dermatitis (atopic dermatitis)*

Natrum mur.	6x
Kali.mur.	6x
Calc.sulph.	6x

d. *Eczema*

Natrum mur.	6x
Natrum sulph.	6x
Kali sulph.	6x

e. *Hair dyes*

Natrum sulph.	6x
Kali.sulph.	6x
Calc.sulph.	6x

f. *Pruritus (itching of skin)*

Kali.mur.	6x
Kali.sulph.	6x
Calc.sulph.	6x

g. *Urticaria*

Nat.mur.	6x
Nat.sulph.	6x
Kali.mur.	6x

31. Smoke allergy

Natrum mur.	6x
Kali.mur.	6x
Calc.sulph.	6x

32. Spices

Natrum sulph.	6x
Kali sulph.	6x
Calc.sulph.	6x

33. Strawberry urticaria

Natrum mur.	6x
Kali.sulph.	6x
Kali.mur.	6x

34. Sugar allergy
        Kali.mur. 6x
        Kali.sulph. 6x
        Calc.sulph. 6x
35. Wheat allergy
        Calc.phos. 6x
        Natrum mur. 6x
        Kali.mur. 6x

ALONE, *likes or desires to be alone*
        Kali.phos. 6x
        Natrum sulph. 6x
        Kali sulph. 6x

ALOPECIA (hair-falling) (See Ringworm and Syphilis also)
        Kali.phos. 6x
        Natrum sulph. 6x
        Calc.sulph. 6x

ALOPECIA, hair falling in old age
        Natrum mur. 6x
        Kali.sulph. 6x
        Calc.sulph. 6x

ALOPECIA AREATA
        Calc.phos. 6x
        Natrum mur. 6x
        Calc.sulph. 6x

ALTERNATING STATES
1. General formula
        Nat.mur. 6x
        Kali.sulph. 6x
        Calc.sulph. 6x
2. Alternating sides of body, complaints on
        Natrum mur. 6x
        Kali.mur. 6x
        Calc.flor. 6x

3. Contradictory states (laughing alternates by weeping)
   - Nat.mur. 6x
   - Kali.sulph. 6x
   - Calc.sulph. 6x

ALZHEIMER'S DISEASE
   - Kali.phos. 6x
   - Kali.mur. 6x
   - Calc.sulph. 6x

AMAUROSIS (blindness) **(See Blindness & vision)**

AMEBIASIS (Amoebic dysentery)
   - Kali.phos. 6x
   - Natrum sulph. 6x
   - Calc.sulph. 6x

AMELIORATIONS (Factors relieving the symptoms)

1. Air, open, ameliorates (but inside room aggravates)
   - Natrum sulph. 6x
   - Kali.mur. 6x
   - Calc.sulph. 6x

2. Air, cool, must have windows open
   - Kali.phos. 6x
   - Natrum sulph. 6x
   - Calc.sulph. 6x

3. Alone, when
   - Kali.phos. 6x
   - Kali.mur. 6x
   - Calc.sulph. 6x

4. After sleep
   - Natrum mur. 6x
   - Kali.mur. 6x
   - Calc.sulph. 6x

5. Bending double
   - Mag.phos. 6x
   - Kali.mur. 6x
   - Calc.flor. 6x

6. Busy or occupied, when

Natrum mur.	6x	
Kali.sulph.	6x	
Calc.sulph.	6x	

7. Cold

Natrum mur.	6x	
Kali.mur.	6x	
Calc.sulph.	6x	

8. Cold open air

Natrum mur.	6x	
Kali.sulph.	6x	
Calc.sulph.	6x	

9. Cold water

Ferrum phos	6x	
Natrum sulph.	6x	
Calc.sulph.	6x	

10. Comany

Natrum mur.	6x	
Kali.sulph.	6x	
Calc.sulph.	6x	

11. Darkness

Nat.mur.	6x	
Kali.mur.	6x	
Calc.sulph.	6x	

12. Drinks, warm

Natrum sulph.	6x	
Kali.sulph.	6x	
Calc.sulph.	6x	

13. Eating

Natrum mur.	6x	
Kali.mur.	6x	
Calc.sulph.	6x	

14. Excitement

Natrum mur.	6x	
Kali.mur.	6x	
Calc.sulph.	6x	

15. Exercise

Kali.phos.	6x
Natrum sulph.	6x
Calc.sulph.	6x

16. Expectoration

Kali.phos.	6x
Calc.sulph.	6x
Silicea	6x

17. Fanned, being

Natrum mur.	6x
Calc.flor.	6x
Silicea	6x

18. Fasting

Natrum sulph.	6x
Kali.sulph.	6x
Calc.sulph.	6x

19. Feet in ice water

Natrum sulph.	*6x*
Kali.sulph.	*6x*
Calc.sulph.	*6x*

20. Friction, rubbing

Natrum sulph.	6x
Kali.sulph.	6x
Calc.sulph.	6x

21. Gentle motion

Ferrum phos	6x
Mag.phos.	6x
Natrum mur.	6x

22. Head, wrapped up warm

Kali.phos.	6x
Natrum sulph.	6x
Calc.sulph.	6x

23. Heat

Kali.mur.	6x
Kali.sulph.	6x
Calc.sulph.	6x

24. Leaning against something

	Kali.mur.	6x
	Nat.mur.	6x
	Calc.sulph.	6x

25. Lying down

	Kali.sulph.	6x
	Calc.sulph.	6x
	Calc.flor.	6x

26. Lying down, on something hard

	Calc.phos.	6x
	Nat.sulph.	6x
	Calc.flor.	6x

27. Lying on left side

	Ferrum phos	6x
	Natrum sulph.	6x
	Calc.sulph.	6x

28. Lying on painful side

	Silicea	6x
	Kali.sulph.	6x
	Calc.sulph.	6x

29. Lying on right side

	Kali.sulph.	6x
	Calc.sulph.	6x
	Calc.flor.	6x

30. Moist warmth

	Calc.phos.	6x
	Natrum sulph.	6x
	Calc.flor.	6x

31. Motion

	Kali.phos.	6x
	Kali.mur.	6x
	Calc.sulph.	6x

32. Pressure

	Mag.phos.	6x
	Natrum mur.	6x
	Calc.sulph.	6x

33. Purging, loose motions	Kali.phos.	6x
	Natrum sulph.	6x
	Calc.sulph.	6x
34. Rain or rainy season	Natrum mur.	6x
	Kali.sulph.	6x
	Calc.sulph.	6x
35. Rest	Natrum sulph.	6x
	Kali.sulph.	6x
	Calc.sulph.	6x
36. Rubbing	Natrum sulph.	6x
	Kali.sulph.	6x
	Calc.sulph.	6x
37. Room, inside	Nat.mur.	6x
	Natrum sulph.	6x
	Silicea	6x
38. Running	Nat.mur.	6x
	Kali.phos.	6x
	Calc.sulph.	6x
39. Sitting	Kali.phos.	6x
	Natrum sulph.	6x
	Kali.sulph.	6x
40. Sitting, erect	Mag.phos.	6x
	Natrum sulph.	6x
	Calc.sulph.	6x
41. Sneezing	Calc.phos.	6x
	Natrum mur.	6x
	Kali.mur.	6x

75

42. Summer, during	Natrum sulph.	6x
	Calc.sulph.	6x
	Silicea	6x
43. Warm, dry weather	Natrum mur.	6x
	Kali.mur.	6x
	Calc.sulph.	6x
44. Warm room	Calc.phos.	6x
	Nat.phos.	6x
	Kali sulph.	6x
45. Warmth, heat	Natrum mur.	6x
	Kali.mur.	6x
	Calc.flor.	6x
46. Wrapping up the head	Kali.mur.	6x
	Calc.sulph.	6x
	Silicea	6x
47. Weather, dry	Natrum sulph.	6x
	Kali.sulph.	6x
	Calc.sulph.	6x

AMENORRHEA

	Calc.phos.	6x
	Ferrum phos	6x
	Kali.sulph.	6x

AMENORRHEA - CAUSES
1. Anaemia

	Calc.phos.	6x
	Ferrum phos	6x
	Natrum mur.	6x

2. Endocrine glands inactivity or hormone imbalance

	Natrum mur.	6x
	Calc.sulph.	6x
	Calc.flor.	6x

3. Mental shock or psychological trauma

Kali.phos.	6x
Natrum mur.	6x
Calc.sulph.	6x

4. Obesity

Natrum mur.	6x
Calc.sulph.	6x
Calc.flor.	6x

5. Primary amenorrhea (menstruarion never started)

Natrum mur.	6x
Natrum sulph.	6x
Kali.mur.	6x

6. Secondary amenorrhea (stoppage in a woman who had menses before)

Calc.phos.	6x
Ferrum phos	6x
Kali.sulph.	6x

AMERICAN TRYPANOSOMIASIS

Kali.phos.	6x
Natrum sulph.	6x
Kali.sulph.	6x
Calc.sulph.	6x

AMNESIA-Imapired memory (See Memory disorders)

AMOEBIC DYSENTERY (Amoebiasis)

Natrum sulph.	6x
Kali.sulph.	6x
Calc.sulph.	6x

AMYOTROPHIC LATERAL SCLEROSIS (AMLS)

Kali.phos.	6x
Natrum sulph.	6x
Calc.sulph.	6x

ANAEMIA
General Formula

Ferr. phos	6x
Nat. mur	6x
Calc. sulph	6x

ANAEMIA - CAUSES AND TYPES

1. After exhaustiong diseases, like malaria, dengue fever, typhoid, irritable bowel syndrome, dysentery, etc.

    Natrum mur.   6x
    Kali.mur.   6x
    Calc.sulph.   6x

2. Excessive menstruation

    Natrum mur.   6x
    Kali.sulph.   6x
    Calc.sulph.   6x

3. From nutritional disturbances

    Kali.sulph.   6x
    Calc.sulph.   6x
    Calc.flor.   6x

5. Blood loss from stomach or duodenal ulcer

    Natrum mur.   6x
    Natrum sulph.   6x
    Kali.mur.   6x

6. Blood loss from piles, over a long period

    Kali.mur.   6x
    Kali.sulph.   6x
    Calc.sulph.   6x

7. Blood loss from kidneys (haematuria)

    Natrum mur.   6x
    Kali.mur.   6x
    Calc.sulph.   6x

8. Bone marrow suppression (aplastic anaemia)

    Natrum mur.   6x
    Kali.mur.   6x
    Calc.sulph.   6x

9. Haemolytic anaemia

    Natrum sulph.   6x
    Kali.sulph.   6x
    Calc.sulph.   6x

10. Iron deficiency anemia

    Ferrum phos   6x
    Natrum mur.   6x
    Silicea   6x

11. Junk foods and processed foods, with preservatives

Kali.sulph.	6x
Calc.sulph.	6x
Calc.flor.	6x

12. Kidney failure

Calc.sulph.	6x
Calc.flor.	6x
Silicea	6x

13. Liver diseases

Natrum mur.	6x
Kali.sulph.	6x
Calc.sulph.	6x

14. Pernicious anaemia

Kali.phos.	6x
Calc.sulph.	6x
Silicea	6x

15. Sickle cell anameia

Kali.sulph.	6x
Calc.sulph.	6x
Calc.flor.	6x

16. Spleen disorders

Natrum mur.	6x
Natrum sulph.	6x
Kali.mur.	6x

17. Thalassemia

Natrum mur.	6x
Kali.mur.	6x
Calc.sulph.	6x

18. Vital drains (blood, catarrh, diabetes, semen, albumin)

Kali.sulph.	6x
Calc.sulph.	6x
Calc.flor.	6x

19. Worms, intestinal (See worms)

ANAL ABSCESS (See Anus, Abscess)

ANAL FISSURE (See Anus)

ANALGESIA (Inability to feel pain or loss of pain sensation)

1. Nerve lesions, neuropathy

Kali.sulph.	6x
Calc.sulph.	6x
Calc.flor.	6x

2. Brain lesions, due to

Kali.phos.	6x
Natrum sulph.	6x
Kali sulph.	6x

3. Spinal cord disorders

Kali.sulph.	6x
Calc.sulph.	6x
Silicea	6x

ANASARCA *(oedema of whole body)* (*See Dropsy also*)

1. General formula for all types of oedema

Nat.mur.	6x
Nat.sulph.	6x
Calc.sulph.	6x

2. Due to heart disease

Kali.phos.	6x
Natrum mur.	6x
Kali.mur.	6x

3. Due to kidney disease

Kali.sulph.	6x
Calc.sulph.	6x
Silicea	6x

4. Due to liver disease

Natrum sulph.	6x
Kali.sulph.	6x
Calc.sulph.	6x

5. Due to nephrotic syndrome

Kali.sulph.	6x
Calc.sulph.	6x
Calc.flor.	6x

6. Due to severe protein deficiency

    Natrum sulph. 6x
    Kali.sulph. 6x
    Calc.sulph. 6x

ANEURYSM

    Calc.flor. 6x
    Kali.sulph. 6x
    Calc.sulph. 6x
    Natrum mur. 6x

ANGER, vexation, irritability

1. Genera formula

    Natrum sulph. 6x
    Kali.sulph. 6x
    Calc.sulph. 6x

2. Abusive language, with

    Natrum mur. 6x
    Natrum sulph. 6x
    Calc.sulph. 6x

3. Ailments, after anger

    Kali.phos. 6x
    Natrum mur. 6x
    Calc.sulph. 6x

4. Ailments, after anger due to Silent grief or indignation

    Nat.mur. 6x
    Kali.mur. 6x
    Calc.sulph. 6x

5. Barks, shouts loudly

    Kali.phos. 6x
    Kali.sulph. 6x
    Calc.sulph. 6x

6. Beats himself

    Natrum mur. 6x
    Natrum sulph. 6x
    Kali.mur. 6x

7. Beats others

    Kali.sulph. 6x
    Calc.sulph. 6x
    Calc.flor. 6x

8. Consolation, aggravates
      Nat.mur. 6x
      Kali.sulph. 6x
      Calc.sulph. 6x

9. Contradiction, from
      Kali.phos. 6x
      Natrum mur. 6x
      Calc.sulph. 6x

10. Can not speak due to anger
      Kali.phos. 6x
      Natrum mur. 6x
      Calc.sulph. 6x

11. Fights with family members only
      Natrum mur. 6x
      Natrum sulph. 6x
      Calc.sulph. 6x

12. Fights with others
      Natrum mur. 6x
      Natrum sulph. 6x
      Kali.sulph. 6x

13. Fits of anger
      Kali.sulph. 6x
      Calc.sulph. 6x
      Calc.flor. 6x

14. Ill-humor, irritabile, cross
      Kali.sulph. 6x
      Calc.sulph. 6x
      Calc.flor. 6x

15. Minor things, from
      Nat.mur. 6x
      Natrum sulph. 6x
      Calc.sulph. 6x

16. Strikes head against the walls or floor
        Kali.phos. 6x
        Mag.phos. 6x
        Nat.phos. 6x

17. Trembling, with violent anger
        Natrum mur. 6x
        Kali.mur. 6x
        Calc.sulph. 6x

18. Violent anger, breaking things, tears clothes
        Kali.sulph. 6x
        Calc.sulph. 6x
        Calc.flor. 6x

ANGINA PECTORIS (pain in heart)
1. Due to poor oxygen supply (ischemia) to the heart muscle
 a. Mag. phos. 6x, repeat after every 15 minutes
 b.   Kali.sulph. 6x
        Calc.sulph. 6x
        Calc.flor. 6x

2. Due to thrombosis or increased clotting of blood
        Natrum sulph. 6x
        Kali.sulph. 6x
        Calc.sulph. 6x

3. Due to coronary arteriosclerosis
        Calc.sulph. 6x
        Kali.sulph. 6x
        Natrum sulph. 6x

ANGIO-NEUROTIC OEDEMA, Anaphylactic shock
        Natrum sulph. 6x
        Kali.mur. 6x
        Calc.sulph. 6x

ANIDROSIS (absence of sweating)
        Kali.phos. 6x
        Kali.mur. 6x
        Calc.sulph. 6x

ANKLES
1. General formula

Kali.mur.	6x
Kali.sulph.	6x
Calc.sulph.	6x

2. Dislocated or turned easily

Kali.sulph.	6x
Calc.sulph.	6x
Calc.flor.	6x

3. Oedema

Natrum sulph.	6x
Kali.sulph.	6x
Calc.sulph.	6x

4. Pain in ankle joint

Natrum mur.	6x
Natrum sulph.	6x
Calc.sulph.	6x

5. Swelling of ankle

Kali.sulph.	6x
Calc.sulph.	6x
Calc.flor.	6x

6. Weak ankle, lame, tendency to easy sprain or dislocation

Kali.phos.	6x
Natrum mur.	6x
Kali.mur.	6x

ANKYLOSING SPONDYLITIS

Kali.phos.	6x
Kali.sulph.	6x
Calc.sulph.	6x

ANKYLOSTOMA DUODENALE

Kali.phos.	6x
Kali.sulph.	6x
Calc.sulph.	6x
Silicea	6x

ANOREXIA NERVOSA

Kali.sulph.	6x
Calc.sulph.	6x
Calc.flor.	6x

ANOSMIA (Loss of sense of smell)

Natrum mur.	6x
Kali.mur.	6x
Silicea	6x

ANSWER, aversion to

Kali.phos.	6x
Natrum mur.	6x
Kali sulph.	6x

ANTHRAX

Natrum sulph.	6x
Kali.sulph.	6x
Calc.sulph.	6x
Silicea	6x

ANTIBIOTIC RESISTANT INFECTIONS

Kali.sulph.	6x
Calc.sulph.	6x
Silicea	6x

ANTIDOTE TO POISONS AND DETOX

Kali.phos.	6x
Natrum sulph.	6x
Silicea	6x

ANTS, as if crawling on parts

Natrum mur.	6x
Kali.mur.	6x
Calc.sulph.	6x

ANXIETY, free floating anxiety or situational anxiety

Calc.phos.	6x
Kali.phos.	6x
Natrum mur.	6x

ANXIETY
1. General formula

Kali.phos.	6x
Natrum sulph.	6x
Calc.sulph.	6x

2. Before menses
- Kali.phos. 6x
- Natrum mur. 6x
- Calc.sulph. 6x

3. During menses
- Kali.sulph. 6x
- Calc.sulph. 6x
- Calc.flor. 6x

4. Fear, with
- Natrum sulph. 6x
- Kali.sulph. 6x
- Calc.sulph. 6x

5. Guilty conscious (as if committed a crime)
- Kali.mur. 6x
- Kali.sulph. 6x
- Calc.sulph. 6x

6. Trifles or small things, about
- Kali.mur. 6x
- Calc.sulph. 6x
- Calc.flor. 6x

ANXIETY NEUROSIS
- Kali.phos. 6x
- Natrum sulph. 6x
- Calc.flor. 6x

ANTHRAX
- Calc.sulph. 6x
- Silicea 6x

ANUS

1. General formula
- Kali.sulph. 6x
- Calc.sulph. 6x
- Silicea 6x

2. Abscess, painful
- Natrum mur. 6x
- Natrum sulph. 6x
- Calc.sulph. 6x

3. Bleeding from anus

Natrum sulph.	6x
Kali.mur.	6x
Kali sulph.	6x

4. Burning in anus

Kali.sulph.	6x
Calc.sulph.	6x
Silicea	6x

5. Burrowing abscess/Peri-anal abscess

Kali.sulph.	6x
Calc.sulph.	6x
Natrum mur.	6x

6. Constriction or narrow anus

Kali.sulph.	6x
Calc.sulph.	6x
Calc.flor.	6x

7. Discharge from anus

Natrum sulph.	6x
Kali.sulph.	6x
Calc.sulph.	6x

8. Excoriation and chaps of anus

Kali.sulph.	6x
Calc.sulph.	6x
Silicea	6x

9. Fissure or cracks in anus

Kali.sulph.	6x
Calc.sulph.	6x
Silicea	6x

10. Fistula of anus

Calc.phos.	6x
Calc.sulph.	6x
Silicea	6x

11. Herpetic eruptions, around anus

Kali.sulph.	6x
Calc.sulph.	6x
Silicea	6x

12. Incontinence of anus
- Kali.mur. 6x
- Kali.sulph. 6x
- Calc.sulph. 6x

13. Irritation in anus
- Kali.sulph. 6x
- Calc.sulph. 6x
- Silicea 6x

14. Itching in anus
- Kali.sulph. 6x
- Calc.sulph. 6x
- Calc.flor. 6x

15. Itching in anus, aggravated at night
- Kali.sulph. 6x
- Calc.sulph. 6x
- Silicea 6x

16. Neuralgia in anus
- Kali.mur. 6x
- Kali.sulph. 6x
- Calc.sulph. 6x

17. Open-anus
- Calc.sulph. 6x
- Calc.flor. 6x
- Silicea 6x

18. Pain (soreness) in anus
- Calc.sulph. 6x
- Kali.sulph. 6x
- Kali.mur. 6x

19. Prolapse of anus
- Kali.sulph. 6x
- Calc.sulph. 6x
- Calc.flor. 6x

20. Rawness of anus
- Kali.sulph. 6x
- Calc.sulph. 6x
- Calc.flor. 6x

21. Wart-like eruptions on anus
    Nat.mur. 6x
    Natrum sulph. 6x
    Kali.sulph. 6x

APATHY (See indifference)
    Kali.phos. 6x
    Natrum sulph. 6x
    Calc.sulph. 6x

APHASIA (Loss of speech due to diseas or injury to brain)
    Kali.phos. 6x
    Natrum mur. 6x
    Calc.sulph. 6x

APHONIA (Loss of voice due to disease of larynx)
    Kali.sulph. 6x
    Calc.sulph. 6x
    Calc.flor. 6x

APHTHOUS ULCERS
    Nat.mur. 6x
    Natrum.sulh. 6x
    Kali.sulph. 6x
    Calc.sulph. 6x

APNOEA (stoppage of breathing, during sleep)
    Kali.phos. 3x
    Kali.sulph. 3x
    Natrum sulph. 3x

APOPLEXY, CEREBRAL (STROKE)
1. General fromul
    Kali.sulph. 6x
    Calc.sulph. 6x
    Calc.flor. 6x
2. Tendeny, to apoplexy
    Kali.phos. 6x
    Natrum mur. 6x
    Kali sulph. 6x

APPENDICITIS

Calc.sulph.	6x
Calc.flor.	6x
Silicea	6x

APPETITE

1. Constant, insatiable appetite

Kali.sulph.	6x
Calc.sulph.	6x
Calc.flor.	6x

2. Easy satiety

Kali.sulph.	6x
Calc.sulph.	6x
Calc.flor.	6x

3. Good appetite, eating well, but with loss of weight

Nat.mur.	6x
Kali.mur.	6x
Calc.sulph.	6x

4. Good appetite with marasmus (atrophy of children)

Natrum mur.	6x
Kali.mur.	6x
Calc.sulph.	6x

5. Good appetite but appetite lost after eating few morsals

Kali.mur.	6x
Kali.sulph.	6x
Calc.sulph.	6x

6. Hungry even after a meal (Bulimia)

Kali.phos.	6x
Kali.sulph.	6x
Calc.sulph.	6x

7. Loss of appetite (see Anorexia also)

Kali.sulph.	6x
Calc.sulph.	6x
Calc.flor.	6x

8. Poor appetite

Natrum mur.	6x
Natrum sulph.	6x
Kali.mur.	6x

APPETITE - PERVERTED, CRAVINGS AND PICA
Excessive Desires

1. Acids, pickles, sour things
   - Natrum mur. 6x
   - Natrum sulph. 6x
   - Kali.mur. 6x
2. Beer
   - Kali.sulph. 6x
   - Calc.sulph. 6x
   - Silicea 6x
3. Butter
   - Kali.sulph. 6x
   - Calc.flor. 6x
   - Silicea 6x
4. Charcoal, coal, chalk, earth, wood, plaster, etc.
   - Calc.phos. 6x
   - Ferrum phos 6x
   - Silicea 6x
5. Coffee
   - Kali.mur. 6x
   - Kali.sulph. 6x
   - Calc.sulph. 6x
6. Drinks, cold
   - Natrum sulph. 6x
   - Kali.sulph. 6x
   - Calc.flor. 6x
7. Drinks, hot
   - Kali.sulph. 6x
   - Calc.sulph. 6x
   - Silicea 6x
8. Effervescent beverages
   - Natrum mur. 6x
   - Kali.mur. 6x
   - Calc.sulph. 6x
9. Eggs
   - Kali.mur. 6x
   - Calc.sulph. 6x
   - Silicea 6x

10. Fats	Natrum sulph.	6x
	Kali.sulph.	6x
	Silicea	6x
11. Lemonade	Natrum sulph.	6x
	Kali.sulph.	6x
	Calc.sulph.	6x
12. Meat	Calc.phos.	6x
	Natrum mur.	6x
	Calc.flor.	6x
13. Salt	Natrum mur.	6x
	Calc.sulph.	6x
	Silicea	6x
14. Sweets, candy	Kali.sulph.	6x
	Calc.sulph.	6x
	Calc.flor.	6x
15. Tea	Calc.sulph.	6x
	Calc.flor.	6x
	Silicea	6x
16. Tobacco	Kali.sulph.	6x
	Calc.sulph.	6x
	Calc.flor.	6x

APPREHESIVENESS (anxiety before an event)

Kali sulph.	6x
Calc.sulph.	6x
Calc.flor.	6x

ARMS

1. Cracking, in joints of arm
   - Calc.sulph. 6x
   - Natrum mur. 6x
   - Kali.sulph. 6x
2. Deltoid muscle, pain or weakness
   - Kali.sulph. 6x
   - Kali.mur. 6x
   - Calc.sulph. 6x
3. Dislocation easy, of joints of arm
   - Kali.mur. 6x
   - Natrum sulph. 6x
   - Kali.sulph. 6x
4. Elbow joint, swelling
   - Calc.sulph. 6x
   - Kali.sulph. 6x
   - Kali.mur. 6x
5. Elbow joint-pain (also see golfer's elbow and tennis elbow)
   - Calc.sulph. 6x
   - Kali.sulph. 6x
   - Kali.mur. 6x
6. Emaciation (atrophy or thinning) of arms
   - Calc.sulph. 6x
   - Kali.sulph. 6x
   - Nat.mur. 6x
7. Eruptions, boils, eczema, herpes, pustules on arms
   - Natrum sulph. 6x
   - Kali.sulph. 6x
   - Calc.sulph. 6x
8. Exostosis (outgrowth, spur of bones), in arm
   - Kali.phos. 6x
   - Calc.sulph. 6x
   - Calc.flor. 6x

9. Feeling of exhaustion or loss of power in arms
  - Kali.mur. 6x
  - Kali.sulph. 6x
  - Calc.sulph. 6x

10. Forearm *(See Forearm)*

11. Heaviness of arms
  - Kali.phos. 6x
  - Nat.mur. 6x
  - Natrum sulph. 6x

12. Motion of arms, convulsive
  - Kali.phos. 6x
  - Kali.mur. 6x
  - Kali sulph. 6x

13. Nodes in arms
  - Calc.flor. 6x
  - Kali.sulph. 6x
  - Calc.sulph. 6x

14. Numbness of arms
  - Kali.phos. 6x
  - Kali.phos. 6x
  - Kali.sulph. 6x
  - Calc.sulph. 6x

15. Numbness, arms and legs
  - Nat.mur. 6x
  - Nat.sulph. 6x
  - Calc.sulph. 6x

16. Pain in arms
  - Kali.mur. 6x
  - Kali.sulph. 6x
  - Clc.phos. 6x

17. Pain in arms while playing piano, violin; typing, sewing, writing
  - Kali.sulph. 6x
  - Calc.sulph. 6x
  - Calc.flor. 6x

18. Pain in arms-raising up the arm

    Calc.flor.   6x
    Kali.sulph.   6x
    Calc.sulph.   6x

19. Pain in arm, ameliorated by
   a. *Rest*

    Kali.sulph.   6x
    Calc.sulph.   6x
    Calc.flor.   6x

   b. *Warmth*

    Kali.phos.   6x
    Natrum sulph. 6x
    Kali.sulph.   6x

20. *Pain in joints of arms (arthritis)*

    Natrum mur.   6x
    Natrum sulph. 6x
    Calc.sulph.   6x

21. Pain in muscles of arms

    Natrum mur.   6x
    Natrum sulph. 6x
    Kali.mur.   6x

22. Paralysis or weakness of forearm

    Kali.mur.   6x
    Kali.sulph.   6x
    Calc.sulph.   6x

23. Paralysis of arm

    Kali.sulph.   6x
    Calc.sulph.   6x
    Calc.flor.   6x

24. Raise the arm, cannot

    Kali.phos.   6x
    Natrum mur.   6x
    Calc.sulph.   6x

25. Suppleness (lack of muscular tone)

    Kali.phos.   6x
    Calc.sulph.   6x
    Silicea   6x

26. Swelling of arm
- Natrum mur. 6x
- Kali.mur. 6x
- Calc.sulph. 6x

27. Swelling in arm-due to vaccination or injection abscess
- Kali.mur. 6x
- Calc.sulph. 6x
- Silicea 6x

28. Trembling of arms
- Kali.phos. 6x
- Natrum sulph. 6x
- Calc.sulph. 6x

29. Weakness of arm
- Kali.phos. 6x
- Natrum sulph. 6x
- Calc.sulph. 6x

30. Weakness of joints of arms
- Kali.phos. 6x
- Mag.phos. 6x
- Calc.sulph. 6x

31. Weakness of arms-sudden
- Natrum mur. 6x
- Natrum mur. 6x
- Calc.sulph. 6x

ARM-PIT (See Axilla)

ARRHYTHMIAS, CARDIAC
- Kali.sulph. 6x
- Calc.sulph. 6x
- Calc.flor. 6x

ARROGANCE (Pride)
- Kali.phos. 6x
- Natrum sulph. 6x
- Calc.sulph. 6x

ARTERIES
1. Atheroma, arteriosclerosis

Kali.sulph.	6x
Calc.sulph.	6x
Calc.flor.	6x

2. Throbbing, pulsating

Natrum mur.	6x
Calc.sulph.	6x
Silicea	6x

3. Thrombosis, embolism

Natrum sulph.	6x
Kali sulph.	6x
Calc.sulph.	6x

ARTERIOSCLEROSIS (See Atherosclerosis)

ARTHRITIS
1. General formula

Ferrum phos	6x
Natrum mur.	6x
Kali.sulph.	6x
Calc.sulph.	6x

2. Large joints- *(Osteo-arthritis)*

Kali.phos.	6x
Natrum mur.	6x
Natrum sulph.	6x
Calc.sulph.	6x

3. Smal joints- (*Rheumatoid arthritis*)

Calc.phos.	6x
Kali.phos.	6x
Natrum sulph.	6x
Calc.sulph.	6x

4. Childhood arthritis

Kali.sulph.	6x
Calc.sulph.	6x
Silicea	6x

5. Fibromyalgia

      Natrum sulph. 6x
      Kali.sulph.   6x
      Calc.sulph.   6x

ARTHRITIS-CHRONIC

      Natrum mur.   6x
      Kali.mur.   6x
      Kali.sulph.   6x
      Calc.sulph.   6x

ARTHRITIS, CHRONIC, with deformities of joints

      Ferrum phos 6x
      Mag.phos.   6x
      Kali.mur.   6x
      Calc.sulph.   6x

ARTHRITIS

1. Ankle joint, arthritis   Calc.phos.   6x
             Mag.phos.   6x
             Calc.sulph.   6x

2. Big toe joint
      Natrum sulph. 6x
      Kali.sulph.   6x
      Calc.sulph.   6x

3. Elbow joint
      Calc.phos.   6x
      Natrum sulph. 6x
      Kali sulph.   6x

4. Finger joints
      Natrum sulph. 6x
      Kali.sulph.   6x
      Calc.sulph.   6x

5. Hip joint
      Natrum sulph. 6x
      Kali.sulph.   6x
      Calc.sulph.   6x
      Silicea   6x

6. Knee joint
     Natrum sulph. 6x
     Kali.sulph. 6x
     Calc.flor. 6x

7. Metacarpo-phalyngeal joints
     Kali.sulph. 6x
     Calc.sulph. 6x
     Silicea 6x

8. Sacro-iliac joints
     Natrum sulph. 6x
     Kali.sulph. 6x
     Calc.sulph. 6x

9. Shoulder joint (frozen shoulder)
     Kali.phos. 6x
     Natrum sulph. 6x
     Kali sulph. 6x

10. Temporo-mandibular joint (TMJ)
     Kali.phos. 6x
     Kali.sulph. 6x
     Calc.sulph. 6x

11. Toes, of foot
     Kali.phos. 6x
     Kali.mur. 6x
     Calc.sulph. 6x

12. Vertebral joints (intervertebral joints) and Disc
     Calc.sulph. 6x
     Kali.mur. 6x
     Calc.sulph. 6x
     Silicea 6x

13. Wrist joint
     Kali.phos. 6x
     Natrum sulph. 6x
     Kali.sulph. 6x
     Calc.sulph. 6x

(See Costochondritis, Osteochondritis also)

ARTHRITIS-*Aggravated by*:
1. Exertion or fatigue or motion
   - Kali.sulph.   6x
   - Calc.sulph.   6x
   - Calc.flor.   6x
2. Night
   - Natrum mur.   6x
   - Natrum sulph.   6x
   - Calc.sulph.   6x

ARTHRITIS-Ameliorated by warmth
   - Mag.phos.   6x
   - Kali.mur.   6x
   - Calc.sulph.   6x

ASCARIS LUMBRICOIDES (ASCARIASIS-Roundworm)
   - Natrum mur.   6x
   - Natrum sulph.   6x
   - Calc.sulph.   6x

(See Worms also)

ASCENDING, aggravates
   - Kali.sulph.   6x
   - Calc.sulph.   6x
   - Calc.flor.   6x

ASCITES
1. General remedy
   - Kali.sulph.   6x
   - Calc.sulph.   6x
   - Calc.flor.   6x
2. Cancer of liver, with
   - Natrum mur.   6x
   - Kali.sulph.   6x
   - Calc.sulph.   6x
3. Cirrhosis of liver, with
   - Natrum mur.   6x
   - Natrum sulph.   6x
   - Kali.sulph.   6x

4. Heart disease or failure, with
   - Mag.phos. 6x
   - Nat.phos. 6x
   - Natrum mur. 6x
5. Jaundice, with
   - Natrum sulph. 6x
   - Kali.sulph. 6x
   - Calc.sulph. 6x
6. Hepatitis, with
   - Mag.phos. 6x
   - Nat.phos. 6x
   - Natrum sulph. 6x

(See Oedema also)

ASPHYXIA (difficult breathing and low oxygen in blood)
1. General formula
   - Kali.sulph. 6x
   - Calc.sulph. 6x
   - Calc.flor. 6x
2. Asphyxia Neonatorum (in newborn)
   - Kali.sulph. 6x
   - Calc.sulph. 6x
   - Calc.flor. 6x

ASTHENOPIA (weakness of eyes) *(See Eyes, Amblyopia)*
   - Natrum mur. 6x
   - Kali.phos. 6x
   - Calc.flor. 6x

ASTHMA-BRONCHIAL *(See Dyspnoea also)*
1. General formula
   - Ferrum phos 6x
   - Natrum mur. 6x
   - Kali.mur. 6x

2. Alternating with eczema

Natrum mur.	6x
Kali.mur.	6x
Calc.flor.	6x

3. Children

Calc.phos.	6x
Kali.phos.	6x
Natrum sulph.	6x

4. Aggravation of asthma by:
   a. *Air, cold*

Natrum mur.	6x
Kali.sulph.	6x
Calc.sulph.	6x

   b. *Ascending, stairs*

Ferrum phos	6x
Natrum sulph.	6x
Calc.flor.	6x

   c. *Change of season*

Natrum sulph.	6x
Kali.sulph.	6x
Calc.sulph.	6x

   d. *Cold weather*

Kali.sulph.	6x
Calc.sulph.	6x
Calc.flor.	6x

   e. *Damp weather*

Natrum mur.	6x
Kali.mur.	6x
Calc.flor.	6x

   f. *Eating food*

Kali.phos.	6x
Calc.sulph.	6x
Calc.flor.	6x

   g. *Exertion*

Natrum mur.	6x
Kali.mur.	6x
Calc.sulph.	6x

h. Heat, hot weather

    Nat.phos. 6x
    Mag.phos. 6x
    Kali.phos. 6x

i. Lying down

    Natrum mur. 6x
    Kali.mur. 6x
    Calc.flor. 6x

j. Night

    Kali.phos. 6x
    Nat.sulph. 6x
    Kali.mur. 6x

k. Winter

    Nat.mur. 6x
    Kali.mur. 6x
    Calc.sulph. 6x

ASTHMA-CAUSED BY

1. Anger

    Kali.phos. 6x
    Natrum mur. 6x
    Calc.sulph. 6x

2. Flatulence

    Natrum mur. 6x
    Kali.mur. 6x
    Calc.flor. 6x

3. Hay asthma or hay fever (Allergic asthma)

    Kali.phos. 6x
    Kali.mur. 6x
    Calc.sulph. 6x

4. Sour foods and drinks

    Kali.mur. 6x
    Kali.sulph. 6x
    Calc.sulph. 6x

5. Nervous causes or emotions

    Nat.mur. 6x
    Kali.phos. 6x
    Kali.sulph. 6x

6. Sycotic constitution

    Nat.sulph. 6x
    Kali sulph. 6x
    Calc.sulph. 6x

7. Thunderstorm, during

    Natrum mur. 6x
    Kali.mur. 6x
    Calc.sulph. 6x

ASTHMA-WITH

1. Bronchial catarrh

    Kali.mur. 6x
    Kali.sulph. 6x
    Calc.sulph. 6x

2. Coryza

    Natrum mur. 6x
    Kali.mur. 6x
    Calc.sulph. 6x

3. Cough

    Calc.phos. 6x
    Nat.mur. 6x
    Kali.mur. 6x

4. Eructations

    Natrum sulph. 6x
    Kali.sulph. 6x
    Calc.sulph. 6x

5. Expectoration, difficult

    Kali.phos. 6x
    Natrum mur. 6x
    Kali.mur. 6x

6. Flatulence

    Kali.mur. 6x
    Kali.sulph. 6x
    Calc.sulph. 6x

7. Fever

    Kali.mur. 6x
    Kali.sulph. 6x
    Calc.sulph. 6x

8. Gastric disorders
   - Kali.phos. 6x
   - Ferrum phos 6x
   - Calc.phos. 6x

ASTHMA - ALLERGIC
1. General formula
   - Natrum mur. 6x
   - Kali.mur. 6x
   - Calc.flor. 6x
2. Birds, parrots; pets like cat, dog, from
   - Natrum sulph. 6x
   - Kali.sulph. 6x
   - Calc.sulph. 6x
3. Dust
   - Calc.phos. 6x
   - Ferrum phos 6x
   - Natrum sulph. 6x
4. Insects
   - Kali.phos. 6x
   - Natrum mur. 6x
   - Calc.flor. 6x
5. Perfumes
   - Kali.mur. 6x
   - Calc.flor. 6x
   - Silicea 6x
6. Pollen
   - Kali.phos. 6x
   - Natrum sulph. 6x
   - Calc.sulph. 6x
7. Smoke
   - Kali.sulph. 6x
   - Calc.sulph. 6x
   - Silicea 6x
8. Tension, anxiety
   - Natrum mur. 6x
   - Kali.sulph. 6x
   - Calc.sulph. 6x

ASTHMA - CARDIAC (Due to heart diseases)

Kali.mur.	6x
Kali sulph.	6x
Calc.sulph.	6x

ASTIGMATISM

Natrum mur.	6x
Kali.sulph.	6x
Calc.sulph.	6x

ATAXIA   See Locomotor ataxia

ATHEROSCLEROSIS

Natrum mur.	6x
Kali.mur.	6x
Calc.sulph.	6x

ATHLETE'S FOOT (Tinea pedis-fungal skin infection of foot which first appears between the toes)

Mag.phos.	6x
Nat.phos.	6x
Natrum sulph.	6x

(See Foot also)

ATOPIC DERMATITIS (Redness & itching of skin-eczema)

Natrum mur.	6x
Calc.sulph.	6x
Silicea	6x

ATHEROMA (Deposition of fats, cholesterol and calcium on the internal walls of arteries)

Natrum mur.	6x
Kali.mur.	6x
Calc.sulph.	6x

ATROPHY (wasting)
1. Arms

Natrum mur.	6x
Natrum sulph.	6x
Kali sulph.	6x

2. Arm, right

Natrum mur.	6x
Kali.mur.	6x
Kali sulph.	6x

3. Arm, left
- Natrum mur. 6x
- Kali.mur. 6x
- Calc.sulph. 6x

4. Body
- Natrum sulph. 6x
- Kali.sulph. 6x
- Calc.sulph. 6x

5. Legs
- Natrum mur. 6x
- Kali.mur. 6x
- Calc.flor. 6x

6. Mammary glands, atrophy, in females
- Natrum mur. 6x
- Kali.mur. 6x
- Calc.sulph. 6x

7. Testes
- Calc.sulph. 6x
- Kali.sulph. 6x
- Natrum sulph. 6x

(See Emaciation and Marasmus also)

ATTENTION, also for patients of attention deficit disorder

Difficult to fix, attention deficit or difficulty in thinking
- Natrum mur. 6x
- Calc.flor. 6x
- Silicea 6x

ATTENTION DEFICIT HYPERACTIVITY DISORDER (ADHD)   (See Mental disorders also)

1. Attention deficit, lack of attention
- Kali.sulph. 6x
- Calc.sulph. 6x
- Silicea 6x

2. Hyperactivity
   - Natrum mur. 6x
   - Kali.sulph. 6x
   - Calc.sulph. 6x
3. Idiotic behvior, disoriented, not oriented in time, place and person
   - Kali.phos. 6x
   - Calc.sulph. 6x
   - Calc.flor. 6x
4. Impulsive, abrupt behavior
   - Calc.phos. 6x
   - Calc.sulph. 6x
   - Calc.flor. 6x
5. Insomnia or sleeplessness
   - Calc.phos. 6x
   - Calc. sulph. 6x
   - Kali.sulph. 6x
6. Lack of control on defecation and urination
   - Natrum mur.
   - Natrum sulph.
   - Kali.mur.
7. Learning (reading and writing) delayed
   - Kali.mur. 6x
   - Kali.sulph. 6x
   - Calc.sulph. 6x
8. Learning, not capable of
   - Natrum mur. 6x
   - Natrum sulph. 6x
   - Kali.mur. 6x
9. No eye contact
   - Kali.mur. 6x
   - Natrum sulph. 6x
   - Natrum mur. 6x
10. No socializtion
   - Kali.mur. 6x
   - Kali.sulph. 6x
   - Calc.sulph. 6x

11. Speech, delayed
	Natrum mur.	6x
	Natrum sulph.	6x
	Calc.flor.	6x

12. Walking, delayed
	Kali.mur.	6x
	Kali.sulph.	6x
	Calc.sulph.	6x

13. Speech and walking, both delayed
	Kali.phos.	6x
	Kali.mur.	6x
	Calc.sulph.	6x

14. Tics   *(See tics)*

15. Toilet training, no learning or delayed learning
	Calc.sulph.	6x
	Calc.flor.	6x
	Silicea	6x

ATTITUDE, bizarre
	Kali.phos.	6x
	Natrum mur.	6x
	Calc.flor.	6x

ATONY OF

1. Bladder (See bladder also)
	Kali.phos.	6x
	Natrum mur.	6x
	Calc.flor.	6x

2. Muscles of body
	Natrum mur.	6x
	Kali.mur.	6x
	Calc.sulph.	6x

AUTISM (ASD-autism spectrum disorders)
(See Mental disorders also)
1. Anger outbursts and irritable behavior
   - Kali.sulph. 6x
   - Calc.sulph. 6x
   - Calc.flor. 6x
2. Concentration problems, lack of focus
   - Kali.mur. 6x
   - Kali.sulph. 6x
   - Calc.sulph. 6x
3. Diarrhea
   - Natrum mur. 6x
   - Natrum sulph. 6x
   - Calc.sulph. 6x
4. Food allergies and digestion problems
   - Natrum sulph. 6x
   - Kali.sulph. 6x
   - Calc.sulph. 6x
5. Hyperactivity, restlessness
   - Calc.sulph. 6x
   - Calc.flor. 6x
   - Silicea 6x
6. Idiotic, senseless behavior (lack of orientation in time, place and person)
   - Natrum mur. 6x
   - Kali.sulph. 6x
   - Calc.sulph. 6x
7. Impulsive or aggressive behavior
   - Natrum mur. 6x
   - Natrum sulph. 6x
   - Kali.mur. 6x
8. Lack of eye contact
   - Kali.sulph. 6x
   - Calc.sulph. 6x
   - Silicea 6x

9. Lack of socialization
    Kali.mur. 6x
    Kali.sulph. 6x
    Calc.sulph. 6x
10. Learning disability or difficulty
    Kali.phos. 6x
    Kali.sulph. 6x
    Calc.sulph. 6x
11. Milk, lactose intolerance
    Natrum sulph. 6x
    Calc.sulph. 6x
    Silicea 6x
12. Sleeplessness
    Natrum mur. 6x
    Kali.mur. 6x
    Calc.sulph. 6x
13. Speech disorders: difficulty or delay in learning speech
    Kali.phos. 6x
    Natrum mur. 6x
    Natrum sulph. 6x
14. Vaccination, ill-effects of
    Kali.phos. 6x
    Natrum mur. 6x
    Calc.sulph. 6x
15. Wheat intolerance
    Kali.sulph. 6x
    Calc.sulph. 6x
    Silicea 6x

AVERSIONS (Dislikes)
1. Acidic foods and drinks
    Ferrum phos 6x
    Natrum mur. 6x
    Calc.sulph. 6x

2. Alcoholic drinks
   - Natrum mur. 6x
   - Kali.mur. 6x
   - Calc.flor. 6x
3. Answer, to
   - Kali.phos. 6x
   - Natrum mur. 6x
   - Kali sulph. 6x
4. Bathing
   - Natrum mur. 6x
   - Kali.sulph. 6x
   - Calc.sulph. 6x
5. Boiled food
   - Kali.sulph. 6x
   - Calc.sulph. 6x
   - Calc.flor. 6x
6. Bread
   - Nat.mur. 6x
   - Kali.mur.. 6x
   - Calc.sulph. 6x
7. Bread and butter
   - Kali.mur. 6x
   - Kali.sulph. 6x
   - Calc.sulph. 6x
8. Butter
   - Nat.sulph. 6x
   - Kali.sulph. 6x
   - Calc.flor. 6x
9. Coffee
   - Kali.mur. 6x
   - Kali.sulph. 6x
   - Calc.sulph. 6x
10. Company
    - Natrum sulph. 6x
    - Kali.mur. 6x
    - Kali.sulph. 6x

11. Drinks, hot	Natrum mur.	6x
	Kali.sulph.	6x
	Calc.sulph.	6x
12. Eggs	Calc.sulph.	6x
	Calc.flor.	6x
	Silicea	6x
13. Fats or fatty foods	Kali.mur.	6x
	Kali.sulph.	6x
	Calc.sulph.	6x
14. Family members	Kali.phos.	6x
	Natrum mur.	6x
	Natrum sulph.	6x
	Calc.flor.	6x
15. Females	Kali.phos.	6x
	Natrum sulph.	6x
	Calc.sulph.	6x
16. Fish	Natrum mur.	6x
	Kali.sulph.	6x
	Calc.sulph.	6x
17. Food	Natrum sulph.	6x
	Kali.mur.	6x
	Kali.sulph.	6x
18. Food, salty	Kali.sulph.	6x
	Calc.flor.	6x
	Silicea	6x
19. Herrings	Natrum mur.	6x
	Natrum sulph.	6x
	Kali.mur.	6x

20. Hot drinks	Natrum mur.	6x
	Kali.sulph.	6x
	Calc.sulph.	6x
21. Hot or warm food	Natrum sulph.	6x
	Kali.sulph.	6x
	Calc.sulph.	6x
22. Husband	Kali.phos.	6x
	Natrum mur.	6x
	Kali.mur.	6x
23. Meat	Natrum sulph.	6x
	Kali.sulph.	6x
	Calc.sulph.	6x
24. Men	Natrum mur.	6x
	Kali.mur.	6x
	Calc.sulph.	6x
25. Milk	Calc.phos.	6x
	Kali.phos.	6x
	Natrum mur.	6x
26. Milk of mother	Kali.sulph.	6x
	Calc.sulph.	6x
	Calc.flor.	6x
27. Motion	Kali.phos.	6x
	Natrum mur.	6x
	Kali sulph.	6x
28. Reading	Kali.phos.	6x
	Kali.mur.	6x
	Silicea	6x

29. School
- Calc.phos. 6x
- Ferrum phos 6x
- Natrum mur. 6x

30. Sour food
- Kali.mur. 6x
- Kali.sulph. 6x
- Calc.sulph. 6x

31. Spices
- Calc.sulph. 6x
- Calc.flor. 6x
- Silicea 6x

32. Spoken, to be
- Kali.phos. 6x
- Natrum sulph. 6x
- Calc.sulph. 6x

33. Sweets
- Kali.sulph. 6x
- Calc.sulph. 6x
- Silicea 6x

34. Tobacco
- Calc.phos. 6x
- Kali.mur. 6x
- Calc.sulph. 6x

35. Tobacco smoking (smoker develops aversion)
- Nat.mur. 6x
- Natrum sulph. 6x
- Kali.mur. 6x

36. Touched, being
- Kali.sulph. 6x
- Calc.sulph. 6x
- Silicea 6x

37. Water or cold water
- Kali.sulph. 6x
- Calc.sulph. 6x
- Calc.flor. 6x

38. Wife
    - Calc.phos. 6x
    - Natrum sulph. 6x
    - Calc.sulph. 6x

39. Wine
    - Natrum mur. 6x
    - Kali.mur. 6x
    - Calc.flor. 6x

40. Women
    - Kali.sulph. 6x
    - Calc.sulph. 6x
    - Silicea 6x

41. Work
    - Kali.sulph. 6x
    - Calc.sulph. 6x
    - Calc.flor. 6x

42. Work, mental
    - Nat.mur. 6x
    - Kali.sulph. 6x
    - Calc.sulph. 6x

(See Foods-that disagree also)

AVIAN INFLUENZA (Bird flu) (See Flu also)
- Kali.phos. 6x
- Natrum sulph. 6x
- Calc.sulph. 6x

AWAKES, screaming
- Kali.phos. 6x
- Natrum mur. 6x
- Kali.mur. 6x

AWAKENED by flatulent pain
- Kali.mur. 6x
- Kali.sulph. 6x
- Calc.sulph. 6x

AWKWARDNESS
1. General formula
    - Kali.phos. 6x
    - Nat.mur. 6x
    - Calc.sulph. 6x

2. Drops things, from hands
   - Kali.phos. 6x
   - Nat.mur. 6x
   - Calc.sulph. 6x
3. Knocks against things while walking
   - Kali.phos. 6x
   - Nat.sulph. 6x
   - Kali.sulph. 6x
4. Stumbles, while walking
   - Nat.mur. 6x
   - Kali.sulph. 6x
   - Calc.sulph. 6x

AXILLA

1. General formula for axillary disease
   - Nat.mur. 6x
   - Natrum sulph. 6x
   - Kali.mur 6x
2. Abscess, boils, acne
   - Kali.phos. 6x
   - Nat.phos. 6x
   - Natrum mur. 6x
3. Eczema
   - Natrum sulph. 6x
   - Kali.sulph. 6x
   - Calc.sulph. 6x
4. Glands (lymph nodes), swelling
   - Kali.mur. 6x
   - Kali.sulph. 6x
   - Calc.sulph. 6x

   See Adenitis also
5. Herpes
   - Natrum mur. 6x
   - Natrum sulph. 6x
   - Calc.sulph. 6x

6. Sweating, excessive
 - Natrum mur. 6x
 - Natrum sulph. 6x
 - Kali.mur. 6x

7. Sweating, offensive, bad smelling
 - Kali.sulph. 6x
 - Calc.sulph. 6x
 - Silicea 6x

8. Sweating, garlic or onion like
 - Calc.sulph. 6x
 - Calc.flor. 6x
 - Silicea 6x

B

BACKACHE-TYPES

1. General formula

Calc.phos.	6x
Kali.phos.	6x
Nat.mur.	6x

2. Aching as if it would break and give out

Kali.phos.	6x
Natrum mur.	6x
Calc.flor.	6x

3. Broken, as if

Kali.phos.	6x
Natrum mur.	6x
Kali.mur.	6x

4. Between scapulae (interscapular region)

Calc.phos.	6x
Kali.phos.	6x
Kali sulph.	6x

5. Bruised type of pain

Kali.mur.	6x
Kali.sulph.	6x
Calc.sulph.	6x

6. Lancinating, drawing, tearing pain

Kali.sulph.	6x
Calc.sulph.	6x
Silicea	6x

7. Lancinating pain, extends down thighs, legs

Calc.phos.	6x
Natrum mur.	6x
Kali sulph.	6x

8. Paralytic pain

Kali.phos.	6x
Natrum mur.	6x
Kali.mur.	6x

9. Radiates to both legs

Kali.sulph.	6x
Calc.sulph.	6x
Silicea	6x

10. Radiates to left leg

Calc.sulph.	6x
Calc.flor.	6x
Silicea	6x

11. Radiates to right leg

Natrum sulph.	6x
Kali.sulph.	6x
Calc.sulph.	6x

BACKACHE - CAUSES

1. Caries of vertebrae, from

Calc.phos.	6x
Calc.flor.	6x
Silicea	6x

2. Crick or sprain in back

Calc.sulph.	6x
Calc.flor.	6x
Silicea	6x

3. Injury or fall, effects of

Kali.phos.	6x
Natrum mur.	6x
Kali sulph.	6x

4. Lifting or overlifting a weight

Kali.sulph.	6x
Calc.sulph.	6x
Calc.flor.	6x

5. Nursing or feeding mothers

Natrum mur.	6x
Natrum sulph.	6x
Kali.mur.	6x

6. Pregnancy

Kali.phos.	6x
Kali.mur.	6x
Calc.sulph.	6x

7. Sexual excesses, from
   - Kali.sulph. 6x
   - Calc.sulph. 6x
   - Calc.flor. 6x
8. Stiffness or spasm of back
   - Mag.phos. 6x
   - Natrum mur. 6x
   - Natrum sulph. 6x
9. Uterine disease, with
   - Natrum sulph. 6x
   - Kali.sulph. 6x
   - Calc.sulph. 6x
10. Vertebral disc degeneration or herniation
    - Kali.phos. 6x
    - Natrum mur. 6x
    - Kali.mur. 6x
11. Vertebral (intervertebral) space, reduction
    - Kali.sulph. 6x
    - Calc.sulph. 6x
    - Calc.flor. 6x
12. Weakness of back
    - Kali.sulph. 6x
    - Calc.sulph. 6x
    - Silicea 6x

BACKACHE - *Aggravation or increases - by:*
1. Bending backward
   - Kali.mur. 6x
   - Kali.sulph. 6x
   - Calc.sulph. 6x
2. Bending forward or stooping
   - Kali.sulph. 6x
   - Calc.sulph. 6x
   - Silicea 6x
3. Coition
   - Kali.phos. 6x
   - Natrum mur. 6x
   - Kali.mur. 6x

4. Exertion
- Natrum mur. 6x
- Natrum sulph. 6x
- Kali.mur. 6x

5. Lifting or overlifting a weight
- Kali.sulph. 6x
- Calc.sulph. 6x
- Calc.flor. 6x

6. Menses, before
- Mag.phos.
- Natrum mur.
- Natrum sulph. 6x

7. Menses, during
- Kali.phos. 6x
- Mag.phos. 6x
- Nat.phos. 6x

8. Motion, walking
- Kali.phos. 6x
- Mag.phos. 6x
- Nat.phos. 6x

9. Night
- Natrum mur. 6x
- Kali.mur. 6x
- Calc.sulph. 6x

10. Pressure
- Kali.sulph. 6x
- Calc.sulph. 6x
- Calc.flor. 6x

11. Rest
- Natrum mur. 6x
- Kali.mur. 6x
- Ferrum phos 6x

12. Riding
- Kali.sulph. 6x
- Calc.flor. 6x
- Calc.sulph. 6x

13. Rising from bed
    - Kali.sulph. 6x
    - Calc.sulph. 6x
    - Calc.flor. 6x
14. Rising from sitting position
    - Kali.sulph. 6x
    - Calc.sulph. 6x
    - Calc.flor. 6x
15. Sitting or sitting for long time
    - Kali.phos. 6x
    - Mag.phos. 6x
    - Nat.phos. 6x
16. Standing or standing for long time
    - Kali.sulph. 6x
    - Calc.sulph. 6x
    - Silicea 6x
17. Straightening up
    - Silicea 6x
    - Kali.sulph. 6x
    - *Calc.sulph.* 6x
18. Walking
    - Calc.sulph. 6x
    - Kali.sulph. 6x
    - Silicea 6x

BACKACHE - Amelioration or better - by:

1. Bending backward
   - Kali.phos.   6x
   - Natrum mur.   6x
   - Kali.mur.   6x

2. Lying
   - Kali.sulph.   6x
   - Calc.sulph.   6x
   - Silicea   6x

3. Lying on back
   - Kali.sulph.   6x
   - Calc.sulph.   6x
   - Silicea   6x

4. Lying on left side
   - Natrum sulph.   6x
   - Kali.mur.   6x
   - Kali sulph.   6x

5. Lying on right side
   - Natrum mur.   6x
   - Natrum sulph.   6x
   - Kali.mur.   6x

6. Lying on something hard
   - Natrum mur.   6x
   - Calc.sulph.   6x
   - Calc.flor.   6x

7. Motion, walking
   - Kali.sulph.   6x
   - Calc.sulph.   6x
   - Calc.flor.   6x

8. Pressure
   - Kali.mur.   6x
   - Calc.sulph.   6x
   - Silicea   6x

BACK- WEAKNESS

	Natrum mur.	6x
	Calc.sulph.	6x
	Silicea	6x

BACTEREMIA

	Ferrum phos	6x
	Natrum sulph.	6x
	Calc.sulph.	6x

BAD BREATH (Halitosis)

	Kali.phos.	6x
	Natrum sulph.	6x
	Calc.sulph.	6x

BAD NEWS, ailments from, or aggravation

	Kali.phos	6x
	Natrum mur.	6x
	Calc.sulph.	6x

BAD PART, takes everything in

	Kali.phos.	6x
	Kali.mur.	6x
	Calc.sulph.	6x

BAKER'S CYST (Popliteal cyst)

	Kali.sulph.	6x
	Calc.sulph.	6x
	Silicea	6x

BAKER's ITCH

	Natrum mur.	6x
	Kali.sulph.	6x
	Calc.sulph.	6x

BALL, sensation of a ball rising in throat

	Natrum sulph.	6x
	Kali.sulph.	6x
	Calc.sulph.	6x

BALL, As if a lump stuck in throat or globus hystericus

	Kali.phos.	6x
	Natrum mur.	6x
	Calc.sulph.	6x

BALANITIS (Inflammation of the glans penis).

  Kali.phos. 6x
  Natrum sulph. 6x
  Calc.sulph. 6x
  Kali.sulph. 6x

BALDNESS, in spots, scalp or beard region

  Calc.phos. 6x
  Natrum mur. 6x
  Calc.sulph. 6x

BALDNESS – (males/females)

  Ferrum phos 6x
  Natrum mur. 6x
  Calc.sulph. 6x

BAND, sensation of hoop
1. Around head, etc.

  Kali.phos. 6x
  Nat.mur. 6x
  Calc.phos. 6x

2. Bones, around

  Natrum mur. 6x
  Natrum sulph. 6x
  Kali.mur. 6x

BANDAGED FEELING

  Ferrum phos 6x
  Kali.sulph. 6x
  Calc.sulph. 6x

BANDAGING, ameliorates

  Kali.phos 6x
  Natrum mur. 6x
  Kali.mur. 6x

BARBER'S ITCH

  Kali.phos. 6x
  Natrum mur. 6x
  Natrum sulph. 6x

BARKING, like a dog

	Calc.sulph.	6x
	Kali.phos.	6x
	Silicea	6x

BAROTITIS MEDIA

	Kali.sulph.	6x
	Calc.sulph.	6x
	Silicea	6x

BARTHOLIN ABSCESS

	Calc.phos.	6x
	Kali.sulph.	6x
	Calc.sulph.	6x

BASHFUL (Timidity, shyness)
1. General formula

	Kali.mur.	6x
	Kali.sulph.	6x
	Calc.sulph.	6x

2. Appearing in public

	Kali.sulph.	6x
	Calc.sulph.	6x
	Silicea	6x

BASEDOW'S DISEASE (toxic diffuse goitre)

(See Goitre, and Hyperthyroidism.

BATHING
1. Aversion to or aggravation from

	Kali.mur.	6x
	Kali.sulph.	6x
	Calc.flor.	6x

2. Aggravation from bathing

	Kali.sulph.	6x
	Calc.sulph.	6x
	Silicea	6x

3. Cold water bathing, aggravates
- Natrum mur. 6x
- Kali.sulph. 6x
- Calc.sulph. 6x

4. Cold water bathing, ameliorates
- Calc.phos. 6x
- Nat.mur. 6x
- Kali.mur. 6x

5. Cold water bathing, desire for
- Kali.mur. 6x
- Kali.sulph. 6x
- Calc.sulph. 6x

6. With hot water, ameliorates
- Natrum sulph. 6x
- Kali.sulph. 6x
- Calc.sulph. 6x

7. In the sea, aggravates
- Kali.sulph. 6x
- Nat.mur. 6x
- Calc.sulph. 6x

BEADS-LIKE swellings
- Calc.sulph. 6x
- Calc.flor. 6x
- Silicea 6x

BEARD, falls out
- Kali.mur. 6x
- Kali.sulph. 6x
- Calc.sulph. 6x

BEARING DOWN PAIN (Pressing down pain in pelvis)
- Calc.phos. 6x
- Kali.phos. 6x
- Nat.mur. 6x

BED SORES, PRESSURE ULCERS

Kali.phos.	6x
Natrum mur.	6x
Natrum sulph.	6x

External use: Apply Calc.sulph. 3x, on the sore.

BED-WETTING (See Enuresis and Urination also)

Kali.phos.	6x
Natrum mur.	6x
Kali.mur.	6x

BED

1. Heat of bed, aggravates the symptoms

Natrum mur.	6x
Kali.mur.	6x
Calc.flor.	6x

2. Lying in bed, ameliorates

Natrum sulph.	6x
Kali.sulph.	6x
Calc.flor.	6x

3. Turning over in bed, aggravates

Natrum mur.	6x
Natrum sulph.	6x
Kali.mur.	6x

BEE-STING

1. Bee-sting-treatment

Kali.phos.	6x
Natrum mur.	6x
Calc.sulph.	6x

2. Bee-sting-sensation

Kali.mur.	6x
Kali.sulph.	6x
Calc.sulph.	6x

3. Bee-sting-Causes anaphylactic reaction/shock

Natrum mur.	6x
Natrum sulph.	6x
Kali.mur.	6x

BELCHING (See Dyspepsia)
BELL'S PALSY *(Paralysis of face)*
1. Left side-Bell's palsy
        Kali.phos. 6x
        Natrum mur. 6x
        Kali.mur. 6x
2. Right side-Bell's palsy
        Kali.phos. 6x
        Natrum sulph. 6x
        Calc.sulph. 6x

BENIGN PROSTATE HYPERPLASIA See Prostate

BERI-BERI (Thiamine or Vitamin B1 deficiency)
        Natrum mur. 6x
        Kali.mur. 6x
        Calc.sulph. 6x

BILE DUCTS DISORDERS-inflammation, blockage
        Nat.mur. 6x
        Natrum sulph. 6x
        Kali.mur. 6x

BILIARY CALCULUS See Gall-stones also
        Calc.phos. 6x
        Ferrum phos 6x
        Natrum sulph. 6x

BILIARY COLIC *(pain in gall bladder)*
        Natrum sulph. 6x
        Kali.mur. 6x
        Kali.sulph. 6x
        Calc.sulph. 6x

Indigestion due to disorders of gall bladder/stones
        Kali.sulph. 6x
        Calc.sulph. 6x
        Silicea 6x

BILIOUSNESS
    Kali.phos. 6x
    Natrum sulph. 6x
    Kali sulph. 6x

BIPOLAR DISORDER
    Kali.phos. 6x
    Kali.mur. 6x
    Calc.flor. 6x

BIRD FLU (See Influenza, Cold, Avian influenza also)
    Kali.phos. 6x
    Natrum sulph. 6x
    Calc.sulph. 6x

BITES cheek or tongue, while chewing or talking
    Kali.sulph. 6x
    Natrum mur. 6x
    Calc.sulph.. 6X

BITES, of insects
    Natrum mur. 6x
    Kali.mur. 6x
    Calc.sulph. 6x

External application: Apply *Calc.sulph.* 3x or 6x

BITES-himself or others (See Mental disorders)

BLACK LUNG (Coal workers' pneumoconioses)
    Natrum sulph. 6x
    Kali.sulph. 6x
    Calc.sulph. 6x

BLADDER, DISEASES
  1. *Atony of bladder (see paralysis also)*
    Kali.phos. 6x
    Natrum sulph. 6x
    Calc.sulph. 6x

  2. Calculi in bladder
    Kali.sulph. 6x
    Calc.sulph. 6x
    Silicea 6x

3. Cancer-bladder
   - Natrum sulph. 6x
   - Kali.sulph. 6x
   - Calc.sulph. 6x
4. Cystitis (inflammation of bladder)
   - Kali.sulph. 6x
   - Calc.sulph. 6x
   - Silicea 6x
5. Enuresis (involuntary urination)
   General remedy
   - Calc.phos. 6x
   - Kali.sulph. 6x
   - Calc.sulph. 6x
   a. *Diurnal (day time)*
   - Kali.phos. 6x
   - Kali.sulph. 6x
   - Calc.sulph. 6x
   b. *Nocturnal (during night)*
   - Natrum mur. 6x
   - Natrum sulph. 6x
   - Calc.sulph. 6x
   c. *Weak or paretic sphincter of bladder*
   - Kali.phos. 6x
   - Kali.sulph. 6x
   - Calc.sulph. 6x
6. Haemorrhage
   - Kali.sulph. 6x
   - Calc.sulph. 6x
   - Silicea 6x
7. Inflammation of bladder (Cystitis)-Acute
   - Kali.sulph. 6x
   - Calc.sulph. 6x
   - Silicea 6x
8. Inflammation of bladder-(Cystitis-Chronic)
   - Kali.sulph. 6x
   - Calc.sulph. 6x
   - Calc.flor. 6x

9. Irritable bladder (frequent urination)
   - Natrum sulph. 6x
   - Kali.sulph. 6x
   - Calc.sulph. 6x
10. Irritable bladder (frequent urination), women
    - Kali.phos. 6x
    - Kali.sulph. 6x
    - Calc.sulph. 6x
11. Old age, bladder problems
    - Kali.mur. 6x
    - Kali.sulph. 6x
    - Calc.sulph. 6x
12. Paralysis of bladder (Weakness, inability to retain urine; Dribbling of urine
    - Kali.sulph. 6x
    - Calc.sulph. 6x
    - Silicea 6x

BLADDER-PAIN
1. General formula
   - Kali.phos. 6x
   - Kali.sulph. 6x
   - Calc.sulph. 6x
2. Burning pain
   - Natrum mur. 6x
   - Kali.mur. 6x
   - Calc.sulph. 6x
3. Cutting, stitching pain in bladder
   - Kali.mur. 6x
   - Kali.sulph. 6x
   - Calc.sulph. 6x
4. Neuralgic, spasmodic pain in bladder
   - Kali.sulph. 6x
   - Calc.sulph. 6x
   - Silicea 6x

5. Radiating to spermatic cord-bladder pain
 Calc.phos. 6x
 Natrum sulph. 6x
 Calc.sulph. 6x

BLEEDING (See Hemorrhage also)
1. General formula for bleeding
 Natrum mur. 6x
 Natrum sulph. 6x
 Calc.sulph. 6x
2. Bleeding-aggravates the symptoms
 Kali.sulph. 6x
 Calc.sulph. 6x
 Calc.flor. 6x
3. Bleeding-ameliorates the symptoms
 Calc.sulph. 6x
 Calc.flor. 6x
 Silicea 6x
4. Gushing blood
 Ferrum phos 6x
 Nat.mur. 6x
 Kali sulph. 6x
5. Streaks of blood (lines of blood on stool, catarrh)
 Kali.mur. 6x
 Kali.sulph. 6x
 Calc.sulph. 6x

BLEPHARITIS *(inflammation of margin of eyelids)*
 Kali.mur. 6x
 Kali.sulph. 6x
 Calc.sulph. 6x

(See Eyes also)

BLINDNESS (Amaurosis)   For details, see Vision.
 Kali.phos. 6x
 Natrum mur. 6x
 Natrum sulph. 6x

BLISTERS
1. General formula
   - Ferrum phos   6x
   - Kali.mur.   6x
   - Calc.sulph.   6x

2. Small blisters, on fingers
   - Kali.mur.   6x
   - Kali.sulph.   6x
   - Calc.sulph.   6x

3. Large blisters, on fingers
   - Natrum mur.   6x
   - Kali.mur.   6x
   - Kali sulph.   6x

4. Lips blisters-on or near, due to fever (herpes labialis)
   - Natrum mur.   6x
   - Kali.sulph.   6x
   - Calc.sulph.   6x

BLOOD CLOTTING
1. Clotting of blood, thrombosis (in any part of body)
   - Natrum sulph.   6x
   - Kali.sulph.   6x
   - Calc.sulph.   6x

2. Clots, quickly (clotting time is decreased)
   - Kali.phos.   6x
   - Kali.mur.   6x
   - Kali sulph.   6x

BLOOD DISORGANISATION
- Kali.phos.   6x
- Mag.phos.   6x
- Natrum sulph.   6x

BLOOD

3. Circulation of blood-sluggish
   - Kali.phos. 6x
   - Natrum mur. 6x
   - Calc.sulph. 6x
4. Clotting of blood, thrombosis (in any part of body)
   - Natrum sulph. 6x
   - Kali.sulph. 6x
   - Calc.sulph. 6x
5. Clots, quickly (clotting time is decreased)
   - Kali.phos. 6x
   - Kali.mur. 6x
   - Kali sulph. 6x
6. Does not clot (small wounds bleed for long time)
   - Calc.phos. 6x
   - Kali.phos. 6x
   - Calc.sulph. 6x
7. Cold blood, sensation as if
   - Kali.phos. 6x
   - Kali.mur. 6x
   - Calc.sulph. 6x
8. Defficiency of blood — *See Anaemia*

9. Disorders of blood, remedy
   - Kali.phos. 6x
   - Mag.phos. 6x
   - Nat.phos. 6x
10. Blood Purifier formula
    - Kali.sulph. 6x
    - Calc.sulph. 6x
    - Silicea 6x

11. Blood and lymphatic system disorders

Kali.mur.	6x
Kali.sulph.	6x
Calc.sulph.	6x

BLOOD SEPSIS (Septicemia and toxemia)

Kali.phos.	6x
Natrum mur.	6x
Calc.sulph.	6x

BLOOD VESSLES
1. Contractility or elasticity of blood vessles-to restore

Natrum mur.	6x
Natrum sulph.	6x
Kali.mur.	6x

2. Enlargement and aneurisms of blood vessels

Calc.phos.	6x
Ferrum phos	6x
Calc.flor.	6x

3. Hardness of walls of blood vessels (athreosclerosis)

Natrum mur.	6x
Natrum sulph.	6x
Kali.mur.	6x

4. Thrombo-embolism of blood

Kali.phos.	6x
Natrum mur.	6x
Natrum sulph.	6x

BLOWS, SHOCKS- electric-like

Natrum mur.	6x
Kali.mur.	6x
Calc.sulph.	6x

BLUISH, purple skin, wounds

Kali.sulph.	6x
Calc.sulph.	6x
Silicea	6x

BLUISH COLOR-Skin, lips, tongue (Cyanosis)
       Kali.phos. 6x
       Natrum mur. 6x
       Kali.mur. 6x

BLOOD PRESUURE-High See Hypertension

BLOOD PRESSURE-Low See Hypotension

BODY, *as a whole*
1. Atrophy of body, wasting or weight loss
       Calc.phos. 6x
       Natrum mur. 6x
       Kali sulph. 6x
2. Bruised sore feeling all over body
       Natrum sulph. 6x
       Kali.sulph. 6x
       Calc.sulph. 6x
3. Burning in various parts of body
       Natrum mur. 6x
       Natrum sulph. 6x
       Kali.mur. 6x
4. Coldness of body
       Kali.sulph. 6x
       Calc.sulph. 6x
       Silicea 6x
5. Exhausted, powerless, feeling, in body
       Kali.phos. 6x
       Natrum sulph. 6x
       Calc.sulph. 6x
6. Heaviness, sensation, in body
       Kali.mur. 6x
       Kali.sulph. 6x
       Calc.sulph. 6x
7. Hot to touch or feels too hot-body
       Kali.sulph. 6x
       Calc.sulph. 6x
       Silicea 6x

8. Numb feeling-all over body
 - Kali.phos. 6x
 - Calc.sulph. 6x
 - Silicea 6x

9. Pain all over the body
 - Kali.sulph. 6x
 - Calc.sulph. 6x
 - Calc.flor. 6x

10. Stiffness of body
 - Kali.mur. 6x
 - Calc.sulph. 6x
 - Silicea

11. Swelling of body (see dropsy also)
 - Calc.phos. 6x
 - Ferrum phos 6x
 - Calc.sulph. 6x

12. Trembling of whole body
 - Nat.phos. 6x
 - Natrum sulph. 6x
 - Calc.sulph. 6x

13. Trembling, internal, sensation-of body
 - Natrum mur. 6x
 - Kali.mur. 6x
 - Calc.sulph. 6x

14. Weakness of body
 - Kali.sulph. 6x
 - Calc.sulph. 6x
 - Calc.flor. 6x

BOILS, furuncles (see Abscess also)

1. General formula for boils
 - Kali.sulph. 6x
 - Calc.sulph. 6x
 - Silicea 6x

2. Crops of boils
 - Kali.sulph. 6x
 - Calc.sulph. 6x
 - Calc.flor. 6x

3. Tendency to boils

    Kali.sulph. 6x
    Calc.sulph. 6x
    Silicea 6x

BONE DISEASES

1. General formula for bone diseases

    Calc.sulph. 6x
    Calc.flor. 6x
    Silicea 6x

2. Caries of bones

    Kali.sulph. 6x
    Calc.sulph. 6x
    Silicea 6x

3. Condyles, epiphyses, swollen-bones

    Kali.sulph. 6x
    Calc.sulph. 6x
    Calc.flor. 6x

4. Curvature of bones (Rickets)

    Kali.mur. 6x
    Kali.sulph. 6x
    Calc.sulph. 6x

5. Development of bones, slow

    Calc.phos 6x
    Calc.fluor 6x
    Silicea 6x

6. Enlargement of bones (Acromegaly)

    Kali.mur. 6x
    Kali.sulph. 6x
    Calc.sulph. 6x

7. Exostosis (outgrowth on bones)

    Kali.sulph. 6x
    Calc.sulph. 6x
    Calc.flor. 6x

8. Fracture of bone

    Kali.sulph. 6x
    Calc.sulph. 6x
    Silicea

9. Fracture of bone-slow union
- Kali.sulph.   6x
- Calc.sulph.   6x
- Calc.flor.   6x

10. Inflammation of bones *(osteitis, osteomyelitis)*
- Natrum mur.   6x
- Natrum sulph. 6x
- Kali.mur.   6x

11. Necrosis (death) of bone
- Kali.sulph.   6x
- Calc.sulph.   6x
- Calc.flor.   6x

12. Necrosis (death) of vertebrae
- Calc.sulph.   6x
- Calc.flor.   6x
- Silicea   6x

13. Osteophytes *(abnormal growth of new pieces of bone)*
- Natrum mur.   6x
- Kali.mur.   6x
- Calc.flor.   6x

14. Pain in bones
- Natrum sulph. 6x
- Kali.sulph.   6x
- Calc.sulph.   6x

15. Tuberculosis of bone
- Natrum mur.   6x
- Natrum sulph. 6x
- Kali sulph.   6x

16. Weak bones, easily fractured
- Kali.phos.   6x
- Kali.mur.   6x
- Calc.sulph.   6x

BORING-fingers into
Ear- boring fingers into
      Natrum mur. 6x
      Natrum sulph. 6x
      Kali.mur. 6x
 Nose - boring fingers into
      Kali.mur. 6x
      Kali.sulph. 6x
      Calc.sulph. 6x

BOWEL OBSTRUCTION, INTUSSUSCEPTION
General formula
      Natrum mur. 6x
      Kali.mur. 6x
      Calc.sulph. 6x
Intestinal Obstruction, post-operative
      Natrum sulph. 6x
      Kali.sulph. 6x
      Calc.sulph. 6x

BRACHIALGIA *(See Neuralgia also)*
      Kali.sulph. 6x
      Calc.sulph. 6x
      Calc.flor. 6x

BRADYCARDIA *(Slow pulse)* *(See Pulse)*

BRAIN DISEASES
1. Abscess in brain
      Kali.sulph. 6x
      Calc.sulph. 6x
      Silicea 6x
2. Atrophy of brain (difficult thinking, concentration, weak memory); dementia, Alzheimer's disease
      Kali.phos. 6x
      Natrum mur. 6x
      Kali.mur. 6x

3. Blood vessels of brain-bursting, as if
    Natrum mur.   6x
    Natrum sulph.   6x
    Calc.sulph.   6x

4. Concussion of brain, in head injury
    Kali.phos.   6x
    Natrum sulph.   6x
    Calc.sulph.   6x

5. Haemorrhage in brain
    Natrum mur.   6x
    Natrum sulph.   6x
    Kali.mur.   6x

6. Hydrocephalus-brain (Abnormal and excess collection of fluid in the ventricles of brain)
    Kali.sulph.   6x
    Calc.sulph.   6x
    Silicea   6x

7. Inflammation of protective membranes of brain (Meningitis, aute or chronic)
    Kali.phos.   6x
    Kali.mur.   6x
    Kali.sulph.   6x
    Calc.sulph.   6x

8. Inflammation-Cerebrospinal
    Kali.mur.   6x
    Kali.sulph.   6x
    Calc.sulph.   6x

9. Ischaemia (giddiness, noises in head, weak memory)
    Kali.mur.   6x
    Kali.sulph.   6x
    Calc.sulph.   6x

10. Oedema of brain
    Kali.mur.   6x
    Kali.sulph.   6x
    Calc.sulph.   6x

11. Oedema of brain-due to high altitude
    Kali.sulph. 6x
    Calc.sulph. 6x
    Silicea 6x

12. Sclerosis of brain (degeneration of brain)
    Calc.sulph. 6x
    Calc.flor. 6x
    Silicea 6x

13. Tumors of brain
    Kali.sulph. 6x
    Calc.flor. 6x
    Calc.sulph. 6x

14. Weakness of brain
    (See Brain, ischemia, Brain-fag)

BRAIN - FAG
    Kali.phos. 6x
    Natrum mur. 6x
    Calc.sulph. 6x

BREAK-UP OF A RELATIONSHIP-bad effects of
    Calc.phos. 6x
    Kali.phos. 6x
    Natrum mur. 6x

BREASTS
1. Abscess in breast
    Kali.phos. 6x
    Natrum sulph. 6x
    Kali.sulph. 6x
    Calc.sulph. 6x

2. Absent or scanty milk
    Calc.phos. 6x
    Ferrum phos 6x
    Kali.phos. 6x

3. Cancer-breast
   - Kali.mur. 6x
   - Kali.sulph. 6x
   - Calc.sulph. 6x
   - Silicea 6x
4. Child dislikes the breast-milk
   - Kali.phos. 6x
   - Kali.sulph. 6x
   - Calc.sulph. 6x
5. Enlarged breasts, in women - to reduce the size
   - Calc.sulph. 6x
   - Calc.flor. 6x
   - Silicea 6x
6. Enlarged breasts, in men (gynaecomastia))
   - Natrum sulph. 6x
   - Kali.sulph. 6x
   - Calc.sulph. 6x
7. Fistulous sinuses in breasts
   - Natrum sulph. 6x
   - Kali.sulph. 6x
   - Calc.sulph 6x
8. Hard knots, in breats
   - Kali.sulph. 6x
   - Calc.sulph. 6x
   - Silicea 6x
9. Induration, hardness-breasts
   - Kali.mur. 6x
   - Kali.sulph. 6x
   - Calc.sulph. 6x
10. Inflammation of breasts (Mastitis)
    - Calc.phos. 6x
    - Kali.phos. 6x
    - Natrum mur. 6x
11. Milk in breasts-absent or deficient
    - Ferrum phos 6x
    - Natrum mur. 6x
    - Calc.sulph. 6x

12. Milk of breasts-bad taste
- Kali.sulph. 6x
- Calc.sulph. 6x
- Silicea 6x

13. Milk in breasts, excessive (Galactorrhoea) - to dry the milk
- Kali.sulph. 6x
- Calc.sulph. 6x
- Silicea 6x

14. Nipples of breasts, cracked, ulcers
- Natrum mur. 6x
- Kali.mur. 6x
- Calc.sulph. 6x

15. Nodules in breast
- Kali.sulph. 6x
- Calc.sulph. 6x
- Calc.flor. 6x

16. Tumors in breasts-benign, non-cancerous
- Kali.sulph. 6x
- Calc.sulph. 6x
- Calc.flor. 6x

17. Under-developed breasts, small in females
- Natrum mur. 6x
- Natrum sulph. 6x
- Kali.sulph. 6x
- Calc.sulph. 6x

BREATHING

1. Breath holding spells or fits in children
   - Kali.phos. 6x
   - Kali.mur. 6x
   - Calc.sulph. 6x

2. Breathing stops on going to sleep (Sleep apnoea)
   - Kali.phos. 3x
   - Kali.sulph. 3x
   - Natrum sulph. 3x

3. Catch in breath
- Natrum mur. 6x
- Kali.mur. 6x
- Calc.sulph. 6x

4. Cold breath
- Kali.sulph. 6x
- Calc.sulph. 6x
- Calc.flor. 6x

5. Desire to take deep breath, sighing
- Natrum mur. 6x
- Kali.sulph. 6x
- Calc.sulph. 6x

6. Difficulty in breathing, labored breathing
- Natrum mur. 6x
- Kali.mur. 6x
- Kali sulph. 6x

7. Offensive, bad breath (fetor oris)
- Kali.phos. 6x
- Kali.mur. 6x
- Calc.sulph. 6x

8. Shortness of breath, or breathlessness
- Kali.phos. 6x
- Kali.sulph. 6x
- Calc.flor. 6x

9. Shortness of breath, on going upstairs
- Natrum mur. 6x
- Kali.sulph. 6x
- Calc.sulph. 6x

10. Will not be able to take next breath, as if
- Natrum mur. 6x
- Natrum sulph. 6x
- Kali.mur. 6x

BRIGHT'S DISEASE (See Nephritis also)

Kali.phos.	6x
Natrum sulph.	6x
Calc.sulph.	6x

BROMIDROSIS *(offensive sweat)* *(See Sweat)*

BRONCHIAL CATARRH, tracheitis, bronchitis

Natrum mur.	6x
Kali.mur.	6x
Calc.sulph.	6x

BRONCHIAL ASTHMA (See Asthma also)

Natrum mur.	6x
Natrum sulph.	6x
Kali.mur.	6x

BRONCHIECTASIS

Kali.phos.	6x
Natrum sulph.	6x
Kali sulph.	6x

BRONCHITIS
1. Acute bronchitis

Kali.mur.	6x
Kali.sulph.	6x
Calc.sulph.	6x

2. Chronic bronchitis

Ferrum phos	6x
Natrum sulph.	6x
Kali sulph.	6x

3. Expectoration, catarrh-yellow

Calc.phos.	6x
Natrum mur.	6x
Kali.mur.	6x

4. Infants, children

	Kali.phos.	6x
	Natrum mur.	6x
	Kali.mur.	6x

BRUISES *(See Injuries)*

BRUXISM *(Grinding teeth and clenching of jaws)*

	Kali.phos.	6x
	Calc.sulph.	6x
	Silicea	6x

BUBO

	Natrum mur.	6x
	Natrum sulph.	6x
	Kali.mur.	6x

BULBAR PARALYSIS *(see paralysis also)*

	Kali.phos.	6x
	Natrum mur.	6x
	Natrum sulph.	6x

BUNION, *on big toe*

	Calc.sulph.	6x
	Calc.flor.	6x
	Silicea	6x

BURNING FEET SYNDROME

	Mag.phos.	6x
	Natrum mur.	6x
	Calc.sulph.	6x

BURNS, SCALDS

	Kali.mur.	6x
	Kali.sulph.	6x
	Calc.sulph.	6x

External application: Above formula in 3x, mixed in Vaseline.

BURSITIS (Inflammation of fluid filled, cushions or sacs, located near large joints to prevent friction)

	Natrum sulph.	6x
	Kali.sulph.	6x
	Calc.sulph.	6x

C

CALCANEAL SPUR (Heel spur, outgrowth of heel bone)

Kali.sulph.	6x
Calc.sulph.	6x
Calc.flor.	6x
Silicea	6x

CALCULI
1. Biliary, gall stones (Cholilithiasis)

Calc.phos.	6x
Ferrum phos	6x
Natrum sulph.	6x

2. Renal, gravel (nephrolithiasis) (See Kidney Stone)

CALLOSITIES, CORNS - on soles of foot

Kali.phos.	6x
Natrum sulph.	6x
Calc.sulph.	6x
Silicea	6x

CANCER
1. General formula

    a. Kali.sulph. 6x
       Calc.flor.
       Calc.sulph. 6x

    b.
Kali.phos.	6x
Natrum mur.	6x
Natrum sulph.	6x
Calc.flor.	6x

2. Bone cancer

Kali.mur.	6x
Kali.sulph.	6x
Calc.sulph.	6x

3. Breast cancer

Kali.mur.	6x
Kali.sulph.	6x
Calc.sulph.	6x
Silicea	6x

4. *Colon cancer*

Kali.sulph.	6x
Calc.sulph.	6x
Calc.flor.	6x
Silicea	6x

5. Liver cancer

a.
Kali sulph.	6x
Calc.sulph.	6x
Calc.flor.	6x
Silicea	

b.
Natrum sulph.	6x
Kali.sulph.	6x
Calc.sulph.	6x

6. Lungs cancer

Natrum sulph.	6x
Kali.mur.	6x
Kali.sulph.	6x
Calc.sulph.	6x

7. Ovary cancer

Kali.sulph.	6x
Calc.sulph.	6x
Silicea	6x

8. Pain of cancer-to relieve

Natrum sulph.	6x
Kali.mur.	6x
Calc.sulph.	6x

9. Pancreas cancer
       Kali.sulph. 6x
       Calc.sulph. 6x
       Silicea   6x

10. Rectum cancer
       Kali.mur. 6x
       Kali.sulph. 6x
       Calc.sulph. 6x

11. Stomach cancer
       Kali.mur. 6x
       Kali.sulph. 6x
       Calc.sulph. 6x

12. Thyroid cancer
       Kali.sulph. 6x
       Calc.sulph. 6x
       Silicea   6x

13. Uterus cancer
       Kali.sulph. 6x
       Calc.sulph. 6x
       Calc.flor. 6x
       Silicea   6x

CANDIDIASIS (fungal infection)
1. Mouth (thrush)
       Kali.phos. 6x
       Natrum sulph. 6x
       Calc.sulph. 6x

2. Vaginal candidiasis
       Kali.phos. 6x
       Natrum sulph. 6x
       Kali.sulph. 6x
       Calc.sulph. 6x

CANKER SORES (aphthous ucers inside the mouth)
       Calc.phos. 6x
       Kali.phos. 6x
       Natrum sulph. 6x

CARBON MONOXIDE POISONING

Kali.phos.	6x
Kali.sulph.	6x
Calc.sulph.	6x

Dose: Reapeat after every 5-10 minute, for 2 hours.

CARBUNCLE (clutser of painfull, pus-filled boils under skin)

Kali.sulph.	6x
Calc.sulph.	6x
Silicea	6x

CARDIAC ARRHYTHMIAS

Kali.phos.	6x
Natrum mur.	6x
Calc.sulph.	6x

CARDIAC DROPSY (Oedema feet due to cardiac disease). (See oedema also)

Natrum mur.	6x
Natrum sulph.	6x
Kali.mur.	6x

CARDIOMYOPATHY

Natrum sulph.	6x
Calc.sulph.	6x
Silicea	6x

CARDIAC FAILURE

1. Acute (myocardial infarction)

Calc.sulph.	6x
Kali.sulph.	6x
Natrum sulph.	6x

Dose in emergency: Repeat every 5 -10 minutes.

2. Congestive cardiac failure (CCF)

Kali.mur.	6x
Natrum mur	6x
Calc.sulph.	6x

CARDIAC NEUROSIS

Kali.phos.	6x
Natrum mur.	6x
Kali.mur.	6x

CARDIALGIA (Heartburn or pain in heart region)
- Kali.mur. 6x
- Calc.sulph. 6x
- Silicea 6x

CARDIAC ORIFICE, Contraction, Reflux Oesophagitis
- Kali.mur. 6x
- Kali.sulph. 6x
- Calc.sulph. 6x

CARPEL TUNNEL SYNDROME
- Natrum mur. 6x
- Kali.mur. 6x
- Calc.sulph. 6x

CARTILAGES, perichondritis *(inflammation, pain)*
- Natrum mur. 6x
- Natrum sulph. 6x
- Kali.mur. 6x

CARIES, BONES *(See Bones, Necrosis)*

CATALEPSY
- Natrum mur. 6x
- Kali.mur. 6x
- Calc.sulph. 6x

CATARACT
- Kali.mur. 6x
- Kali.sulph. 6x
- Calc.sulph. 6x

CATARRH, CATARRHAL TROUBLES
- Natrum sulph. 6x
- Kali.sulph. 6x
- Calc.sulph. 6x

CATHETERISM (Urethritis and fever due to catheter)
- Calc.phos. 6x
- Natrum sulph. 6x
- Kali.sulph. 6x
- Calc.sulph. 6x

CAT-SCRATCH DISEASE
    Kali.phos. 6x
    Natrum sulph. 6x
    Kali.sulph. 6x
    Calc.sulph. 6x

CATS – INFECTIONS, FROM
    Kali.phos. 6x
    Natrum sulph. 6x
    Calc.sulph. 6x

CELIAC DISEASE (Wheat allergy, Gluten enteropathy)
    Calc.phos. 6x
    Kali.sulph. 6x
    Calc.sulph. 6x

CELLULITIS (A serious bacterial skin infection)
    Kali.sulph. 6x
    Calc.sulph. 6x
    Silicea 6x

CEREBRAL PALSY (Brain disorder with inability to move and maintain balance)
    Kali.sulph. 6x
    Calc.sulph. 6x
    Silicea

CEREBRO-SPINAL MENINGITIS *(See Meningitis)*

CERVICAL SPONDYLOSIS
    Calc.phos. 6x
    Kali.phos. 6x
    Natrum mur. 6x

CERVICITIS (Inflammation of neck of uterus)
    Kali.phos. 6x
    Natrum sulph. 6x
    Calc.sulph. 6x

CHAFFING OF SKIN, IN FOLDS *OF SKIN*
    Kali.sulph. 6x
    Calc.sulph. 6x
    Calc.flor. 6x

CHALAZION (See Eye)
CHANCRE, Syphilitic
1. Primary lesion-of syphilitic chancre
    - Kali.sulph. 6x
    - Calc.sulph. 6x
    - Calc.flor. 6x
2. Bleeding or phagedenic- syphilitic chancre
    - Kali.sulph. 6x
    - Calc.sulph. 6x
    - Silicea 6x

CHECKED (STOPPED) DISCHARGES, *ill-effects* of
1. General formula
    - Kali.phos. 6x
    - Calc.sulph. 6x
    - Calc.flor. 6x
2. Foot sweats, stopped, ill-effects of
    - Kali.phos. 6x
    - Natrum mur. 6x
    - Kali.mur. 6x
3. Eruptions, suppressed, ill-effects of
    - Natrum sulph. 6x
    - Kali.mur. 6x
    - Kali sulph. 6x

CHEEK, bites cheek or tongue, while chewing or talking
- Kali.phos. 6x
- Natrum mur. 6x
- Calc.sulph. 6x

CHEEKS-Yellow saddle (Lupus)
- Kali.phos. 6x
- Natrum mur. 6x
- Natrum sulph. 6x

CHEILITIS (Inflammation of lips or corners of mouth)
Angular cheilitis (corners of mouth)
- Natrum sulph. 6x
- Calc.sulph. 6x
- Silicea 6x

CHICKEN-POX
        Natrum mur. 6x
        Natrum sulph. 6x
        Kali.mur. 6x
CHILBLAINS-Fingers and toes
        Natrum sulph. 6x
        Kali.sulph. 6x
        Calc.sulph. 6x
CHILD-ABUSE (See Children)
CHILD BIRTH (See Delivery, Labor)
CHILDREN – DISEASES (See Autism, Cough, Tonsils *and other diseases under the respective topics*)
 1. Abuse victims (child abuse victims)
        Natrum sulph. 6x
        Kali.sulph. 6x
        Calc.sulph. 6x
 2. Broken family victims
        Kali.phos. 6x
        Natrum sulph. 6x
        Calc.sulph. 6x
 3. Slow leraning to speak
        Ferrum phos 6x
        Natrum sulph. 6x
        Calc.sulph. 6x
 4. Slow leraning to walk
        Kali.sulph. 6x
        Calc.sulph. 6x
        Silicea 6x
 5. Slow to leran to talk and walk
        Kali.sulph. 6x
        Calc.sulph. 6x
        Silicea 6x

CHILDHOOD ARTHRITIS (See arthritis)
CHILLINESS, Coldness

    Natrum mur.   6x
    Natrum sulph. 6x
    Kali sulph.   6x

CHLOASMA, MELASMA, liver spots, moth patches on cheek

    Ferrum phos   6x
    Natrum mur.   6x
    Natrum sulph. 6x

CHLOROSIS   See Anaemia

CHOLECYSTITIS (Inflammation of gall bladder)

    Natrum sulph. 6x
    Kali.mur.   6x
    Calc.sulph.   6x

CHOLERA

    Natrum mur.   6x
    Natrum sulph. 6x
    Kali.mur.   6x

CHOLERA INFANTUM-Summer Complaint

    Kali.sulph.   6x
    Calc.sulph.   6x
    Silicea   6x

CHOLILITHIASIS (Gall stones)

    Kali.phos.   6x
    Natrum sulph. 6x
    Calc.sulph.   6x

(In emergency repeat after every hour, till the pain subsides)

CHOREA, St Vitus Dance-(involuntary jerky movements)
General remedy

  a. Mag.phos.   6x
      Kali.mur.   6x
      Natrum mur. 6x
  b. Calc.phos.   6x
      Kali.phos.   6x
      Kali sulph.   6x

Chorea-worse during sleep
- Kali.mur. 6x
- Kali.sulph. 6x
- Calc.sulph. 6x

CHRONIC FATIGUE SYNDROME
- Kali.phos. 6x
- Natrum sulph. 6x
- Kali.sulph. 6x
- Calc.sulph. 6x

CIRCUMCISION – (for quick healing of wound)
- Kali.phos. 6x
- Natrum sulph. 6x
- Calc.sulph. 6x

Dose: two doses before and three times daily afterwards.

CHRONIC WASTING DISEASES (Marasmus, tuberculosis, diabetes, autoimmune disease, cancer, kidney and liver failure)
- Kali.phos. 6x
- Natrum sulph. 6x
- Calc.sulph. 6x

CIRRHOSIS, OF LIVER (See Liver also)
- Natrum sulph. 6x
- Kali.sulph. 6x
- Calc.sulph. 6x

CLAIRVOYANCE (perceiving the remote or future events)
- Kali.phos. 6x
- Natrum mur. 6x
- Natrum sulph. 6x

CLAUSTROPHOBIA (Fear of closed spaces)
- Kali.phos. 6x
- Kali.sulph. 6x
- Calc.sulph. 6x

CLERGYMAN'S SORE THROAT-Speakers, teachers
- Calc.sulph. 6x
- Calc.flor. 6x
- Silicea 6x

CLIMACTERIC (Menopause) DISORDERS

1. General formula for climacteric disorders
   - Kali.sulph. 6x
   - Calc.sulph. 6x
   - Silicea 6x
2. Anger, irritability-(during climacteric)
   - Kali.phos. 6x
   - Natrum mur. 6x
   - Kali.mur. 6x
3. Breasts, enlarged, painful: inframammary pain
   - Kali.sulph. 6x
   - Calc.sulph. 6x
   - Silicea 6x
4. Burning, in vertex (top of head), palms and soles
   - Kali.mur. 6x
   - Kali.sulph. 6x
   - Calc.sulph. 6x
5. Depression-(during climacteric)
   - Kali.phos. 6x
   - Natrum mur. 6x
   - Natrum sulph.
6. Fainting spells-(during climacteric)
   - Kali.sulph. 6x
   - Calc.sulph. 6x
   - Calc.flor. 6x
7. Fatigue, weakness, chilliness-(during climacteric)
   - Kali.sulph. 6x
   - Calc.sulph. 6x
   - Silicea 6x
8. Fibroids, in uterus-(during climacteric)
   - Kali.mur. 6x
   - Kali.sulph. 6x
   - Calc.sulph. 6x

9. Flooding (excessive menstruation, metrorrhagia)
   - Calc.sulph. 6x
   - Calc.flor. 6x
   - Silicea 6x
10. Flushing- sudden hot flushes with sweating
    - Kali.phos. 6x
    - Natrum mur. 6x
    - Natrum sulph. 6x
11. Globus hystericus, hysterical tendencies-(climacteric)
    - Natrum mur. 6x
    - Natrum sulph. 6x
    - Kali.mur. 6x
12. Hair-falling-(during climacteric)
    - Natrum mur. 6x
    - Natrum sulph. 6x
    - Kali.mur. 6x
13. Headcahe-(during climacteric)
    - Kali.phos. 6x
    - Natrum mur. 6x
    - Natrum sulph. 6x
14. Jealousy-(during climacteric)
    - Kali.sulph. 6x
    - Calc.flor. 6x
    - Calc.sulph. 6x
15. Pain, inflammation, in uterus-(during climacteric)
    - Kali.mur. 6x
    - Kali.sulph. 6x
    - Calc.sulph. 6x
16. Palpitations-(during climacteric)
    - Kali.phos. 6x
    - Natrum mur. 6x
    - Calc.sulph. 6x
17. Sweating, excessive-(during climacteric)
    - Kali.phos. 6x
    - Kali.mur. 6x
    - Calc.sulph. 6x

CLOTTING OF BLOOD-DECREASED (Bleeding tendency)

Calc.sulph.	3x
Calc. flor.	3x
Silicea	3x

CLOTTING OF BLOOD-INCREASED (Thrombosis)

Kali.sulph.	6x
Kali.mur.	6x
Silicea	6x

COCCYX (Tail bone)

1. Injury, pain in coccyx (Coccygodynia, Coxalgia)

Kali.phos.	6x
Kali.sulph.	6x
Calc.sulph.	6x

2. Itching in coccyx

Kali.phos.	6x
Natrum sulph.	6x
Calc.sulph.	6x

3. Numbness in coccyx

Kali.phos.	6x
Kali.mur.	6x
Calc.sulph.	6x

4. Ulcer-coccyx

Kali.phos.	6x
Kali.mur.	6x
Calc.flor.	6x

COITION (Sexual intercourse)

1. Desire-absent in female

Natrum sulph.	6x
Kali.mur.	6x
Kali sulph.	6x

2. Desire-absent in male

Kali.phos.	6x
Kali.sulph.	6x
Calc.sulph.	6x

3. No ejaculation occurs in male
       Kali.phos. 6x
       Kali.sulph. 6x
       Natrum mur. 6x
4. No pleasure, during coition
       Kali.phos. 6x
       Natrum sulph. 6x
       Calc.sulph. 6x
5. No orgasm occurs in female
       Natrum sulph. 6x
       Kali.sulph. 6x
6. Calc.sulph. Orgasms in female without intercourse
       Kali.phos. 6x
       Calc.sulph. 6x
       Silicea 6x

7. Painful in women (vaginismus)
       Natrum mur. 6x
       Kali.mur. 6x
       Calc.sulph. 6x

COLD (See Commin cold, Flu, Influenza)
COLD SORES (herpes simplex or fever blisters on lips)
       Kali.phos. 6x
       Natrum sulph. 6x
       Calc.sulph. 6x
COLIC (colicky pain in abdominal viscera)
 1. General formula
       Mag.phos. 6x
       Natrum mur. 6x
       Kali.mur. 6x
       Calc.sulph. 6x
 2. Babies-colic
       Kali.sulph. 6x
       Calc.sulph. 6x
       Silicea 6x

3. Biliary colic, (gall-stone colic)
   - Natrum sulph. 6x
   - Kali.sulph. 6x
   - Calc.sulph. 6x
4. Chronic tendency to colic
   - Natrum sulph. 6x
   - Kali.sulph. 6x
   - Calc.sulph. 6x
5. Flatulent colic (colic due to gas)
   - Natrum mur. 6x
   - Natrum sulph. 6x
   - Kali.mur. 6x
6. Hypgastrium-colic (in centre of abdomen below stomach)
   - Kali.sulph. 6x
   - Calc.sulph. 6x
   - Silicea 6x
7. Hysterical causes-colic
   - Natrum mur. 6x
   - Kali.mur. 6x
   - Calc.sulph. 6x
8. Ileo-cecal region-colic
   - Kali.sulph. 6x
   - Calc.sulph. 6x
   - Calc.flor. 6x
9. Intestine, small-colic
   - Kali.mur. 6x
   - Kali.sulph. 6x
   - Calc.sulph. 6x
10. Intestine, large-colic
    - Kali.mur. 6x
    - Kali.sulph. 6x
    - Calc.sulph. 6x

11. Kidney-colic (Renal colic)

Natrum mur.	6x
Natrum sulph.	6x
Kali.mur.	6x

12. Kidney stone colic (Renal stone colic)

Kali.sulph.	6x
Calc.sulph.	6x
Calc.flor.	6x

13. Menstrual colic

Kali.mur.	6x
Kali.sulph.	6x
Calc.sulph.	6x

14. Stomach-colic

Kali.mur.	6x
Kali.sulph.	6x
Calc.sulph.	6x

15. Toxic or poison colic (due to lead or copper)

Mag.phos.	6x
Natrum sulph.	6x
Calc.sulph.	6x

16. Ureteric colic

Ferrum phos	6x
Mag.phos.	6x
Natrum mur.	6x

COLIC - AGGRAVATION

1. Bending forward-increases colic

Kali.phos.	6x
Kali.sulph.	6x
Calc.sulph.	6x

2. Fasting-increases the colic

Kali.phos.	6x
Kali.mur.	6x
Calc.flor.	6x

COLIC - AMELIORATION
1. Bending double - decreases the colic
   - Mag.phos. 6x
   - Kali.sulph. 6x
   - Calc.sulph. 6x
2. Flatus, expelled out-decreases the colic
   - Kali.sulph. 6x
   - Calc.sulph. 6x
   - Calc.flor. 6x
3. Heat or warm application-decreases the colic
   - Kali.phos. 6x
   - Natrum sulph. 6x
   - Kali sulph. 6x

COLITIS (Inflammation of colon mucosa)
- Natrum mur. 6x
- Kali.mur. 6x
- Calc.sulph. 6x

1. Natrum mur. 6x
   - Kali.sulph. 6x
   - Calc.sulph. 6x
   - Silicea 6x

CONCUSSION (Shock to brain due to head injury)
- Kali.phos. 6x
- Natrum sulph. 6x
- Calc.sulph. 6x

CONVULSIONS (See Epilepsy)
COPLEXION-FAIR, to make (See Face)
COPD-(Chronic obstructive pulmonary disease)
- Kali.mur. 6x
- Kali.sulph. 6x
- Calc.sulph. 6x

COLLAPSE (See Weakness)

COLOR-BLINDNESS (See Vision)

COMA

1. General formula
   - Natrum mur. 6x
   - Kali.sulph. 6x
   - Calc.sulph. 6x
2. Brain haemorrhage
   - Kali.phos. 6x
   - Natrum sulph. 6x
   - Calc.sulph. 6x
3. Head injury, concussion
   - Kali.phos. 6x
   - Natrum sulph. 6x
   - Calc.sulph. 6x
4. Liver failure (Hepatic coma)
   - Natrum sulph. 6x
   - Kali.mur. 6x
   - Kali sulph. 6x
5. Low blood pressure
   - Kali.phos. 6x
   - Natrum mur. 6x
   - Kali.mur. 6x
6. Low blood sugar level
   - Natrum mur. 6x
   - Kali.mur. 6x
   - Calc.sulph. 6x

   (Must take Glucose by mouth or by injection as well)
7. High blood sugar level
   - Kali.mur. 6x
   - Kali.sulph. 6x
   - Calc.sulph. 6x
8. Keto-acidosis
   - Kali.phos. 6x
   - Natrum mur. 6x
   - Natrum sulph. 6x

9. Ureamic coma (coma due to increased urea level)

Kali.phos.	6x
Natrum mur.	6x
Kali.sulph.	6x
Calc.sulph.	6x
Silicea	6x

COMEDONES (Black-heads or white-heads)

Calc.phos.	6x
Kali.sulph.	6x
Calc.sulph.	6x

COMMON COLD

1. Acute cold

Natrum sulph.	6x
Kali.sulph.	6x
Calc.sulph.	6x

2. Chronic cold

Natrum mur.	6x
Kali.mur.	6x
Calc.sulph.	6x
Silicea	6x

3. Dry, stuffy colds

Natrum mur.	6x
Kali.mur.	6x
Calc.sulph.	6x

4. Fluent, watery cold

Natrum mur.	6x
Natrum sulph.	6x
Kali.mur.	6x

5. With thick mucus-cold

Kali.sulph.	6x
Calc.sulph.	6x
Silicea	6x

6. Cough, with-cold

Kali.sulph.	6x
Calc.sulph.	6x
Silicea	6x

7. Headache with cold
 - Kali.mur. 6x
 - Calc.sulph. 6x
 - Calc.flor. 6x

8. Hoarseness, aphonia with cold
 - Kali.sulph. 6x
 - Calc.sulph. 6x
 - Silicea 6x

9. Infants, with catarrh
 - Kali.sulph. 6x
 - Calc.sulph. 6x
 - Calc.flor. 6x
 - Silicea 6x

10. Inflammation, chronic, atrophic sicca (Dryness of mucus memebrane of nose)
 - Natrum mur. 6x
 - Kali.mur. 6x
 - Calc.flor. 6x

11. Inflammation, chronic, catarrhal
 - Natrum mur. 6x
 - Kali.mur. 6x
 - Calc.sulph. 6x

12. Recurrent colds/flu
 - Kali.sulph. 6x
 - Calc.sulph. 6x
 - Silicea 6x

13. Sneezing, with cold
 - Natrum sulph. 6x
 - Kali.sulph. 6x
 - Calc.sulph. 6x

COMPLAINTS, SYMPTOMS – TYPES OF

1. Appear, in small spots
 - Kali.sulph. 6x
 - Calc.sulph. 6x
 - Calc.flor. 6x

2. Erratic, shifting, changing symptoms
      Kali.sulph. 6x
      Calc.sulph. 6x
      Silicea 6x
3. From cold or chilling
      Kali.mur. 6x
      Kali.sulph. 6x
      Silicea 6x
4. From, over-lifting the weight, straining, stretching
      Calc.sulph. 6x
      Calc.flor. 6x
      Silicea 6x
5. Symptoms Improve, then relapse continually
      Calc.phos. 6x
      Ferrum phos 6x
      Kali.phos. 6x
6. In old people
      Kali.sulph. 6x
      Calc.sulph. 6x
      Silicea 6x

CONCUSSION (Brain injury, Head injury)
      Kali.phos. 6x
      Natrum sulph. 6x
      Calc.sulph. 6x

CONJUNCTIVITIS (See Eye)

CONDYLOMATA (See Warts)

CONSTIPATION
1. General formula
      Kali.phos. 6x
      Natrum mur. 6x
      Natrum sulph. 6x
2. From inertia and dryness of intestines
      Kali.mur. 6x
      Kali.sulph. 6x
      Silicea 6x

3. Dry, stool
 - Natrum mur. 6x
 - Kali.mur. 6x
 - Calc.sulph. 6x

4. Dry stool, ball or dung-like
 - Kali.mur. 6x
 - Kali.sulph. 6x
 - Calc.sulph. 6x

5. Dry stool, that must be mechanically removed
 - Kali.sulph. 6x
 - Calc.sulph. 6x
 - Calc.flor. 6x

6. Frequent, ineffectual urging, unsatisfactory
 - Kali.phos. 6x
 - Natrum mur. 6x
 - Kali.mur. 6x

7. No desire or urging of stool, for many days
 - Kali.phos. 6x
 - Natrum mur. 6x
 - Kali.mur. 6x
 - Calc.sulph. 6x

8. Soft stool-even passed with difficulty
 - Kali.sulph. 6x
 - Calc.sulph. 6x
 - Calc.flor. 6x

CONSTIPATION - Concomitants

1. With piles
 - Natrum mur. 6x
 - Kali.mur. 6x
 - Calc.sulph. 6x

2. With anal prolapse
 - Natrum sulph. 6x
 - Kali.sulph. 6x
 - Calc.sulph. 6x

3. Rectal pain, persistent, after passing stool
        Natrum mur. 6x
        Kali.mur. 6x
        Kali.sulph. 6x
        Calc.sulph. 6x

CONVALESCENCE (Recovery phase from disease)
        Kali.phos. 6x
        Natrum sulph. 6x
        Calc.sulph. 6x

CONVULSIONS (see Epilepsy also)
1. Clonic convulsions
        Kali.phos. 6x
        Natrum mur. 6x
        Calc.sulph. 6x
2. Isolated group of muscles-convulsions
        Kali.phos. 6x
        Natrum mur. 6x
        Kali.mur. 6x
        Calc.sulph. 6x
3. Puerperal Convulsions
        Natrum sulph. 6x
        Kali.sulph. 6x
        Calc.sulph. 6x
4. Teething, dentition, in children
        Kali.phos. 6x
        Natrum sulph. 6x
        Kali.sulph. 6x
        Calc.sulph. 6x
5. Tonic convulsions
        Natrum sulph. 6x
        Kali.sulph. 6x
        Calc.sulph. 6x
6. Uremic convulsions
        Kali.sulph. 6x
        Calc.sulph. 6x
        Calc.flor. 6x

7. Worms-Convulsions, due to
          Nat.phos.   6x
          Natrum sulph.   6x
          Silicea   6x

CORNEA

1. Abscess
          Natrum sulph.   6x
          Kali.sulph.   6x
          Calc.sulph.   6x

2. Inflammation of cornea (Keratitis)
          Kali.sulph.   6x
          Calc.sulph.   6x
          Silicea   6x

3. Keratoconus
          Kali.phos.   6x
          Natrum sulph.   6x
          Kali sulph.   6x

4. Opacities of cornea
          Calc.phos.   6x
          Kali.mur.   6x
          Calc.sulph.   6x

5. Ulcers of cornea
          Kali.phos.   6x
          Natrum mur.   6x
          Kali.mur.   6x

6. Wounds, injury of cornea with sharp instrument
          Kali.sulph.   6x
          Calc.sulph.   6x
          Silicea   6x

CORN AND CALLOSITIES

          Natrum sulph.   6x
          Kali.sulph.   6x
          Calc.flor.   6x

CORONARY ARTERIES
1. Atherosclerosis, blockage, spasm of coronary artery
   - Kali.phos. 6x
   - Natrum sulph. 6x
   - Calc.sulph. 6x
2. Thrombosis of coronary artery
   - Natrum sulph. 3x
   - Kali.sulph. 6x
   - Calc.sulph. 6x

CORYZA See Commom cold, Flu, Influenza, Catarrh

COSTO-CHONDRITIS (inflammation of the cartilage which joins the ribs with the sternum or central breastbone)
- Natrum sulph. 6x
- Kali.sulph. 6x
- Calc.sulph. 6x

COUGH
1. General formula
   - Natrum mur. 6x
   - Natrum sulph. 6x
   - Kali.mur. 6x
2. Bacterial cough
   - Kali.mur. 6x
   - Kali.sulph. 6x
   - Calc.sulph. 6x
3. Bronchospam or suffocation, with
   - Mag.phos. 6x
   - Nat.phos. 6x
   - Calc.sulph. 6x
4. Cough, fever, dyspnea, shock-leading to death
   - Kali.sulph. 6x
   - Calc.sulph. 6x
   - Silicea 6x

5. Dry cough
   - Natrum mur. 6x
   - Natrum sulph. 6x
   - Kali sulph. 6x

6. Difficulty in breathing, with
   - Natrum mur. 6x
   - Natrum sulph. 6x
   - Calc.sulph. 6x

7. Chronic cough
   - Natrum sulph. 6x
   - Kali.sulph. 6x
   - Calc.sulph. 6x

8. Fever, with
   - Natrum sulph. 6x
   - Kali.mur. 6x
   - Calc.sulph. 6x

9. Fever and chills, with
   - Kali.mur. 6x
   - Kali.sulph. 6x

10. Calc.sulph. Fibrosis of lungs, with
    - Natrum sulph. 6x
    - Calc.flor. 6x
    - Silicea 6x

11. Hoarse, hollow, metallic cough
    - Natrum sulph. 6x
    - Kali.sulph. 6x
    - Calc.sulph. 6x

12. Low oxygen saturation in blood
    - Kali.sulph. 6x
    - Calc.sulph. 6x
    - Silicea 6x

13. Productive cough, with expectoration
    - Natrum sulph. 6x
    - Kali.sulph. 6x
    - Calc.sulph. 6x
    - Silicea 6x
14. Viral cough
    - Kali.sulph. 6x
    - Calc.sulph. 6x
    - Silicea 6x
15. Weakness, extreme, with cough
    - Kali.sulph. 6x
    - Calc.sulph. 6x
    - Calc.flor. 6x
    - Silicea 6x

COWPERITIS
- Ferrum phos 6x
- Natrum sulph. 6x
- Calc.sulph. 6x

CRACKS
1. Lips, cracks and ulceration
    - Natrum mur. 6x
    - Kali.mur. 6x
    - Calc.sulph. 6x
2. Mouth, corners of (angular cheilitis or stomatitis)
    - Calc.phos. 6x
    - Kali.phos. 6x
    - Kali.mur. 6x
3. Skin-cracks
    - Kali.sulph. 6x
    - Calc.sulph. 6x
    - Calc.flor. 6x

CRAMPS
1. General formula
    - Kali.phos. 6x
    - Mag.phos. 6x
    - Calc.sulph. 6x

2. During diarrhea, dehydration and electrolytes loss
   - Kali.phos. 6x
   - Natrum mur. 6x
   - Kali.mur. 6x
3. Feet and toes
   - Kali.sulph. 6x
   - Calc.sulph. 6x
   - Calc.flor. 6x
4. Hands and fingers
   - Mag.phos. 6x
   - Natrum sulph. 6x
   - Calc.sulph. 6x
5. Intestinal muscles-cramps
   - Kali.sulph. 6x
   - Calc.sulph. 6x
   - Calc.flor. 6x
6. Leg muscles-cramps
   - Kali.mur. 6x
   - Kali.sulph. 6x
   - Calc.sulph. 6x
7. Menstrual cramps (cramps and pain during menses)
   - Natrum mur. 6x
   - Natrum sulph. 6x
   - Kali.mur. 6x
8. Preme-menstrual cramps
   - Kali.mur. 6x
   - Kali.sulph. 6x
   - Calc.sulph. 6x

CREATININE-RAISED LEVELS (in kidney failure)
   - Calc.phos. 6x
   - Ferrum phos 6x
   - Calc.sulph. 6x

CRETINISM (physical deformity and learning difficuly due to by birth thyroid dysfunction)

Natrum sulph.	6x
Kali.sulph.	6x
Calc.sulph.	6x

CROHN'S DISEASE (Inflammatory bowel disease)

Kali.phos.	6x
Natrum sulph.	6x
Kali.sulph.	6x
Calc.sulph.	6x

CROUP (inflammation of larynx, trachea and bronchi which obstructs the breathing and causes the barking cough)

Natrum sulph.	6x
Kali.sulph.	6x
Calc.sulph.	6x

CUSHING SYNDROME (Excess production of cortisol)

Calc.sulph.	6x
Natrum sulph.	6x
Kali sulph.	6x

CUTS, CRACKS, IN SKIN

Kali.phos.	6x
Natrum sulph.	6x
Calc.sulph.	6x

CYANOSIS (bluish color of skin, tongue, nails, due to deficiency of oxygen in blood)

Kali.phos.	6x
Mag.phos.	6x
Nat.phos.	6x

CYSTITIS (inflammation of bladder)   See Bladder

CYST - KIDNEY

Natrum mur.	6x
Kali.sulph.	6x
Calc.sulph.	6x

CYSTS - OVARIAN

Kali.phos.	6x
Natrum sulph.	6x
Calc.sulph.	6x

CYSTS-Sebaceous

    Kali.phos.   6x
    Calc.sulph. 6x
    Calc.flor.   6x
    Silicea   6x

CYSTIC TUMORS

    Kali.phos.   6x
    Kali.mur.   6x
    Calc.sulph. 6x
    Silicea   6x

D

DANDRUFF - Scalp, hair

Natrum mur.	6x
Natrum sulph.	6x
Kali.mur.	6x

(See Seborrhoea also). Scaling on scalp and hair is called dandruff and on face and body it is called seborrhea.

DEAFNESS

1. General formulae for all types of deafness

   a. Kali.phos.   6x
   Natrum sulph.   6x
   Calc.sulph.   6x

   b. Ferrum phos.   6x
   Kali. mur.   6x
   Kali. phos.   6x

2. Due to adenoids or enlarged tonsils

   Kali.mur.   6x
   Kali.sulph.   6x
   Calc.sulph.   6x

3. Catarrh, inflammation (eustachean, middle ear)

   Natrum mur.   6x
   Natrum sulph.   6x
   Kali.mur.   6x

4. Head injury, due to

   Kali.sulph.   6x
   Calc.sulph.   6x
   Silicea   6x

5. Hearing loss

   a. Conductive hearing loss

   Kali.phos.   6x
   Kali.mur.   6x
   Calc.sulph.   6x

b. Sensorineural hearing loss
- Kali.mur. 6x
- Kali.sulph. 6x
- Calc.sulph. 6x

c. Mixed hearing loss
- Natrum mur. 6x
- Natrum sulph. 6x
- Kali.mur. 6x

6. Human voice, difficult to hear
- Natrum sulph. 6x
- Kali.mur. 6x
- Kali sulph. 6x

7. Injury to ear by loud sound or blast
- Natrum mur. 6x
- Natrum sulph. 6x
- Kali.mur. 6x

8. Nerve (auditory nerve) defects
- Kali.phos. 6x
- Kali.mur. 6x
- Calc.sulph. 6x

9. Noise, loud, due to
- Calc.sulph. 6x
- Calc.flor. 6x
- Silicea 6x

10. Old age
- Natrum mur. 6x
- Natrum sulph. 6x
- Kali.mur. 6x

11. Scrofulous diathesis
- Kali.mur. 6x
- Kali.sulph. 6x
- Calc.sulph. 6x

12. With tinnitus and/or vertigo
- Kali.sulph. 6x
- Calc.sulph. 6x
- Calc.flor. 6x

13. With vertigo
    Kali.sulph.   6x
    Calc.sulph.   6x
    Silicea   6x

DEBILITY (See Weakness)
DECUBITUS (See Bed Sores)
DEEP VEIN THROMBOSIS (DVT)
    Natrum sulph.   6x
    Calc.sulph.   6x
    Silicea   6x

DEGENERATIVE INERVERTEBRAL DISC DISORDERS
    Kali.mur.   6x
    Kali.sulph.   6x
    Calc.sulph.   6x

DELIRIUM (See Mental disorders)
DELIVERY, EASY (Easy delivery formula)
    Mag.phos.   6x
    Calc.phos   6x
    Kali.phos   6x
    Calc.fluor   6x

Dose: Once daily in seven months and three times daily during last two months of pregnancy.

DEMENTIA (Alzheimer's disease)
    Kali.phos.   6x
    Kali.mur.   6x
    Calc.sulph.   6x

DENGUE FEVER
1. Classical degue fever
    Calc.sulph.   6x
    Kali.phos.   6x
    Natrum sulph.   6x
    Kali.sulph.   6x

2. Dengue hemorrhagic fever without shock
   - Kali.phos. 12x
   - Kali.mur. 12x
   - Calc.sulph. 12x
   - Silicea 12x
3. Dengue hemorrhagic fever with shock
   - Calc.sulph. 12x
   - Kali.sulph. 12x
   - Kali.phos. 12x
   - Natrum sulph. 12x
4. Platelets deficiency in dengue fever
   - Natrum sulph. 6x
   - Kali.mur. 6x
   - Calc.sulph. 6x
5. Weakness after dengue syndrome
   - Kali.phos. 6x
   - Natrum sulph. 6x
   - Kali.sulph. 6x
   - Calc.sulph. 6x

DENTAL ABSCESS (Peri-apical, peri-odontal abscess)
- Ferrum phos 6x
- Kali sulph. 6x
- Calc.sulph. 6x

DENTITION (Teething)
1. Healthy dentition, to promote
   - Calc.phos. 6x
   - Ferrum phos 6x
   - Calc.flor. 6x
2. Teething difficult, delayed, retlessness
   - Nat.phos. 6x
   - Natrum sulph. 6x
   - Calc.sulph. 6x
3. Diarrhea, during dentition
   - Natrum sulph. 6x
   - Kali.sulph. 6x
   - Calc.sulph. 6x

4. Fever during dentition
- Natrum sulph. 6x
- Kali.mur. 6x
- Calc.flor. 6x

5. Irritability and crying during dentition
- Kali.sulph. 6x
- Calc.sulph. 6x
- Silicea 6x

DEPRESSION

1. General formula
   - Kali.phos. 6x
   - Natrum mur. 6x
   - Kali.mur. 6x

2. Neurotic depression (without hallucinations)
   - Kali.phos. 6x
   - Natrum sulph. 6x
   - Calc.sulph. 6x

3. Psychotic deression (with hallucinations)
   - Natrum sulph. 6x
   - Kali.mur. 6x
   - Kali.sulph. 6x

DERMATITIS (Inflammation of skin) (See Skin also)
- Natrum sulph. 6x
- Kali.sulph. 6x
- Calc.sulph. 6x

DERMATOMYOSITIS (inflammation of muscle & skin rash)
- Kali.sulph. 6x
- Calc.sulph. 6x
- Silicea 6x

DERMATOPHYTE INEFECTION (See Ringworm)

DERMOID CYST (Collection of various tissues under skin)
- Calc.phos. 6x
- Calc.sulph. 6x
- Calc.flor. 6x

DESIRES, EXCESSIVE CRAVINGS

1. Alcohol or ale

Calc.phos.	6x
Kali.phos.	6x
Kali.mur.	6x

2. Bacon

Calc.sulph.	6x
Calc.flor.	6x
Silicea	6x

3. Bitter foods

Kali.phos.	6x
Nat.sulph.	6x
Calc.sulph.	6x

4. Cold drinks-carbonated drinks

Kali.sulph.	6x
Calc.sulph.	6x
Silicea	6x

5. Eggs

Calc.phos.	6x
Kali.sulph.	6x
Calc.sulph.	6x

6. Fast foods

Natrum mur.	6x
Natrum sulph.	6x
Kali.mur.	6x

7. Fruit or claret

Natrum mur.	6x
Natrum sulph.	6x
Calc.flor.	6x

8. Green and sour vegetables

Natrum mur.	6x
Kali.mur.	6x
Calc.sulph.	6x

9. Ham

Kali.sulph.	6x
Calc.sulph.	6x
Silicea	6x

10. Indigestible things

Kali.sulph.	6x
Calc.sulph.	6x
Silicea	6x

11. Salted foods

Calc.sulph.	6x
Calc.flor.	6x
Silicea	6x

12. Smoked meat

Kali.sulph.	6x
Calc.sulph.	6x
Silicea	6x

13. Sour articles, pickles

Kali.phos.	6x
Natrum mur.	6x
Kali.mur.	6x

14. Spicy foods

Calc.phos.	6x
Ferrum phos	6x
Natrum sulph.	6x

15. Stimulants

Kali.sulph.	6x
Calc.sulph.	6x
Calc.flor.	6x

16. Sugar, sweets

Kali.sulph.	6x
Calc.sulph.	6x
Silicea	6x

DEVIATED NASAL SEPTUM (DNS)

Natrum sulph.	6x
Kali.sulph.	6x
Calc.sulph.	6x

DIABETES INSIPIDUS

Kali.phos.	6x
Natrum sulph.	6x
Calc.sulph.	6x

DIABETES MELLITUS

1. General formula
   - Kali.sulph. 6x
   - Calc.sulph. 6x
   - Calc.flor. 6x
   - Silicea 6x
2. Non-insulin dependent cases
   - Calc.phos. 6x
   - Ferrum phos 6x
   - Kali.phos. 6x
   - Kali sulph. 6x
3. Insulin dependent cases
   - Kali.sulph. 6x
   - Calc.sulph. 6x
   - Silicea 6x
4. Gestational diabetes (diabetes during pregnancy)
   - Natrum sulph. 6x
   - Kali.mur. 6x
   - Calc.sulph. 6x

DIABETES MELLITUS - CAUSES

1. Autoimmune disorders
   - Natrum mur. 6x
   - Kali.mur. 6x
   - Calc.sulph. 6x
2. Drugs, due to
   - Kali.phos. 6x
   - Natrum mur. 6x
   - Calc.sulph. 6x
3. Endocrine diseases, due to
   - Natrum sulph. 6x
   - Kali.sulph. 6x
   - Calc.sulph. 6x

4. Pancreas infections, due to
   - Calc.sulph. 6x
   - Natrum sulph. 6x
   - Kali sulph. 6x

DIABETES MELLITUS - TYPES

1. Juvenile onset DM (childhood-Insulin dependent)
   - Kali.sulph. 6x
   - Calc.sulph. 6x
   - Silicea 6x
2. Maturity onset DM (adults above 30 years age)
   - Kali.phos. 6x
   - Kali.sulph. 6x
   - Calc.sulph. 6x

DIABETES - COMPLICATIONS

1. Abscess-foot (diabetic foot)
   - Natrum sulph. 6x
   - Kali.sulph. 6x
   - Calc.sulph. 6x
2. Arteriosclerosis
   - Kali.mur. 6x
   - Calc.sulph. 6x
   - Silicea 6x
3. Gangrene-foot
   - Natrum mur. 6x
   - Natrum sulph. 6x
   - Calc.sulph. 6x
4. Heart disorders
   - Kali.sulph. 6x
   - Calc.sulph. 6x
   - Silicea 6x
5. Impotence (males)
   - Kali.phos. 6x
   - Kali.sulph. 6x
   - Silicea
6. Nephropathies (kidney complications)
   - Natrum sulph. 6x
   - Kali.sulph. 6x
   - Calc.sulph. 6x

7. Neuropathies (diabetic neuropathies)
   - Kali.phos. 6x
   - Calc.sulph. 6x
   - Calc.flor. 6x
8. Numbness-due to diabetes
   - Kali.phos. 6x
   - Natrum sulph. 6x
   - Calc.sulph. 6x
9. Retinopathies (due to diabetic) and loss of vision
   - Kali.phos. 6x
   - Mag.phos. 6x
   - Calc.flor. 6x
10. Sex-related problems in males (impotence, etc)
    - Kali.phos. 6x
    - Kali.mur. 6x
    - Calc.sulph. 6x
11. Skin problems-dry, wrinkled-due to dibetes
    - Kali.mur. 6x
    - Kali.sulph. 6x
    - Calc.sulph. 6x
12. Weakness, lethary-due to diabetic
    - Kali.sulph. 6x
    - Calc.sulph. 6x
    - Silicea 6x

DIABETIC FOOT (See Diabetes-complications)
DIABETIC RETINOPATHY (See Diabetes-complications)

DIAPER RASH (Nappy rash)
- Calc.sulph. 6x
- Ferrum phos. 6x
- Kali. sulph. 6x

DIAPER RASH - FUNGAL
- Calc. sulph 6x
- Kali.sulph. 6x
- Natrum.sulph. 6x

DIAPHRAGM (Inflammation, irritation)
        Natrum mur.   6x
        Kali.mur.   6x
        Calc.sulph.   6x

DIARRHOEA - DYSENTERY

1. General formula
        Kali.phos.   6x
        Natrum mur.   6x
        Kali.mur.   6x
        Calc.sulph.   6x

2. From emotional excitement, fright
        Kali.phos.   6x
        Kali.mur.   6x
        Calc.sulph.   6x

3. From fatty foods
        Kali.sulph.   6x
        Calc.sulph.   6x
        Silicea   6x

4. From fruits
        Mag.phos.   6x
        Nat.phos.   6x
        Natrum sulph.   6x

5. From gastric derangements
        Kali.phos.   6x
        Natrum sulph.   6x
        Calc.sulph.   6x

6. From hot weather
        Kali.sulph.   6x
        Calc.sulph.   6x
        Calc.flor.   6x
        Silicea   6x

7. From intestinal atony, debility
        Kali.phos.   6x
        Kali.mur.   6x
        Calc.sulph.   6x

8. From milk

	Kali.phos.	6x
	Natrum sulph.	6x
	Kali sulph.	6x

9. From typhoid fever

	Kali.sulph.	6x
	Calc.sulph.	6x
	Silicea	6x

10. From vegetables, melon

	Kali.sulph.	6x
	Calc.sulph.	6x
	Silicea	6x

11. Infants (dentition) (See Dentition)
12. Old age diarrhea

	Natrum sulph.	6x
	Kali.sulph.	6x
	Calc.flor.	6x

DIARRHOEA - TYPES OF STOOL

1. Bloody diarrhoea

	Ferrum phos	6x
	Natrum mur.	6x
	Kali.mur.	6x

2. Blood streaked, stool

	Natrum sulph.	6x
	Kali.sulph.	6x
	Calc.flor.	6x

3. Debilitating (weakening), diarrhea

	Kali.phos.	6x
	Natrum sulph.	6x
	Calc.sulph.	6x

4. Fermented, flatulent diarrhoea
   - Kali.phos. 6x
   - Natrum sulph. 6x
   - Kali.sulph. 6x
   - Calc.sulph. 6x
5. Gelatinous, jelly-like
   - Mag.phos. 6x
   - Nat.phos. 6x
   - Natrum sulph. 6x
6. Involuntary diarrhea
   - Kali.phos. 6x
   - Kali.mur. 6x
   - Silicea 6x
7. Rice-water diarrhea
   - Natrum sulph. 6x
   - Kali.sulph. 6x
   - Calc.sulph. 6x
8. Sudden diarrhea, cannot wait
   - Kali.sulph. 6x
   - Calc.sulph. 6x
   - Silicea 6x

DIFFUSE TOXIC GOITER
- Natrum mur. 6x
- Kali sulph. 6x
- Calc.sulph. 6x

DIPHTHERIA
- Ferrum phos 6x
- Natrum sulph. 6x
- Kali.sulph. 6x
- Silicea 6x

DIPLOPIA (double vision)   (See Eyes)

DISC - VERTEBRAL, DISORDERS
1. General formula

Natrum mur.	6x
Kali.mur.	6x
Kali.sulph.	6x
Calc.sulph.	6x

2. Bulging, Dgeneration of vertebral disc

Calc.sulph.	6x
Natrum sulph.	6x
Calc.flor.	6x

DIVERTICULITIS (Inflammation in pouches of intestine)

Natrum sulph.	6x
Kali.sulph.	6x
Calc.sulph.	6x

DIZZINESS (See Vertigo also)

Kali.phos.	6x
Natrum sulph.	6x
Calc.sulph.	6x

DROPSY
See Oedema 6x

DROWSINESS
1. General formula

Natrum sulph.	6x
Calc.sulph.	6x
Silicea	6x

2. After meals-drowsiness

Natrum sulph.	6x
Kali.sulph.	6x
Calc.sulph.	6x

3. Diabetic patients-drowsiness

Kali.phos.	6x
Kali.sulph.	6x
Calc.sulph.	6x

DRUGS, DIETS-ABUSE, ill-ffects of

1. General formula for ill-effects of drugs and diets abuse
   - Kali.mur. 6x
   - Kali.sulph. 6x
   - Calc.sulph. 6x
2. Analgesics abuse
   - Kali.phos. 6x
   - Natrum sulph. 6x
   - Calc.sulph. 6x
3. Antibiotics abuse
   - Kali.sulph. 6x
   - Calc.sulph. 6x
   - Silicea 6x
4. Antihistamines abuse
   - Kali.sulph. 6x
   - Calc.sulph. 6x
   - Silicea 6x
5. Chemotherapy for cancer treatment
   - Kali.phos. 6x
   - Natrum sulph. 6x
   - Kali.mur. 6x
   - Kali sulph. 6x
6. Fast foods
   - Natrum sulph. 6x
   - Kali.sulph. 6x
   - Calc.sulph. 6x
7. Fats, fried foods
   - Natrum sulph. 6x
   - Kali.mur. 6x
   - Calc.sulph. 6x
8. Iron abuse
   - Kali.phos. 6x
   - Natrum sulph. 6x
   - Kali sulph. 6x

9. Narcotics abuse

Kali.phos.	6x
Natrum mur.	6x
Kali sulph.	6x

10. Quinine abuse

Kali.phos.	6x
Natrum mur.	6x
Calc.sulph.	6x

11. Radiation exposure or radiation therapy

Kali.mur.	6x
Kali.sulph.	6x
Calc.sulph.	6x

12. Salt intake-excessive

Natrum mur.	6x
Kali.sulph.	6x
Silicea	6x

13. Sedatives abuse

Kali.sulph.	6x
Calc.sulph.	6x
Silicea	6x

14. Spices

Natrum sulph.	6x
Kali.sulph.	6x
Calc.sulph.	6x

15. Steroids

Kali.phos.	6x
Kali.mur.	6x
Calc.sulph.	6x

16. Sugar

Kali.phos.	6x
Natrum sulph.	6x
Calc.sulph.	6x

DRY EYE AND DRY MOUTH (Sjogren's syndrome)

Calc.phos.	6x
Natrum mur.	6x
Kali.mur.	6x

DUBIN JOHNSON SYNDROME (Genetic disease of liver)
Natrum sulph. 6x
Kali sulph. 6x
Calc.sulph. 6x

DUODENUM-Inflammation (Duodenitis) or ulcer
Natrum sulph. 6x
Kali.sulph. 6x
Calc.sulph. 6x

DUPUYTREN'S CONTRACTURE
(See Hands)

DYSENTERY (See Diarrhoea also)
Ferrum phos 6x
Natrum mur. 6x
Kali.mur. 6x

DYSFUNCTIONAL UTERINE BLEEDING
Ferrum phos 6x
Natrum mur. 6x
Calc.sulph. 6x

DYSLEXIA (Learning disability)
Kali.phos. 6x
Natrum sulph. 6x
Calc.sulph. 6x

DYSMENORRHOEA (painful menstruation)
1. General formula
Mag.phos. 6x
Kali.sulph. 6x
Calc.sulph. 6x
Calc.flor. 6x
2. Irregular menses
Calc.flor. 6x
Kali.sulph. 6x
Calc.sulph. 6x
3. Spasmodic pain, with uterine congestion
Kali.phos. 6x
Kali.sulph. 6x
Calc.sulph. 6x

DYSPEPSIA (indigestion, acidity, nausea)-CAUSES

1. General formula
   - a. Natrum sulph. 6x
     - Kali.mur. 6x
     - Calc.sulph. 6x
   - b. Ferrum phos. 6x
     - Kali. mur. 6x
     - Natrum phos. 6x

2. Abuse of drugs, tea, tobacco, condiments
   - Natrum sulph. 6x
   - Kali.sulph. 6x
   - Calc.sulph. 6x

3. Aged, debilitated persons
   - Calc.phos. 6x
   - Kali.phos. 6x
   - Natrum mur. 6x

4. Beer-dyspepsia
   - Natrum mur. 6x
   - Natrum sulph. 6x
   - Calc.sulph. 6x

5. Dietetic indiscretions-dyspepsia
   - Ferrum phos 6x
   - Nat.phos. 6x
   - Natrum sulph. 6x

6. Excesses (over eating, excessive sex)-dyspepsia
   - Kali.phos. 6x
   - Kali.mur. 6x
   - Calc.sulph. 6x

7. Fatty food-dyspepsia
   - Natrum sulph. 6x
   - Calc.sulph. 6x
   - Silicea 6x

8. Flatulent food-dyspepsia
   - Natrum sulph. 6x
   - Calc.sulph. 6x
   - Silicea 6x
9. Milk-dyspepsia
   - Kali.phos. 6x
   - Natrum sulph. 6x
   - Kali sulph. 6x
10. Sedentary life style - -dyspepsia
    - Natrum sulph. 6x
    - Kali.sulph. 6x
    - Calc.sulph. 6x
11. Tea-dyspepsia
    - Natrum sulph. 6x
    - Calc.flor. 6x
    - Silicea 6x
12. Tobacco-dyspepsia
    - Nat.phos. 6x
    - Calc.sulph. 6x
    - Silicea 6x

DYSPEPSIA-SYMPTOMS
1. Acidity
   - Nat.phos. 6x
   - Natrum sulph. 6x
   - Calc.sulph. 6x
2. Digestion, weak, slow
   - Kali.phos. 6x
   - Kali.mur. 6x
   - Calc.sulph. 6x
3. Distress from simplest food
   - Natrum sulph. 6x
   - Kali.sulph. 6x
   - Calc.sulph. 6x

4. Eructations, excessive and loud
    - Calc.sulph. 6x
    - Kali.sulph. 6x
    - Natrum sulph. 6x
5. Eructations, foul
    - Natrum sulph. 6x
    - Kali.sulph. 6x
    - Calc.sulph. 6x
6. Flatulent distention of stomach
    - Natrum sulph. 6x
    - Calc.sulph. 6x
    - Silicea 6x
7. Heartburn, pyrosis
    - Kali.phos. 6x
    - Natrum sulph. 6x
    - Calc.sulph. 6x
8. Nausea, Vomiting
    - Natrum sulph. 6x
    - Kali.sulph. 6x
    - Calc.sulph. 6x
9. Pain, immediately after eating
    - Natrum sulph. 6x
    - Calc.sulph. 6x
    - Silicea 6x
10. Pain, several hours after eating
    - Natrum sulph. 6x
    - Kali.sulph. 6x
    - Calc.flor. 6x
11. Palpitation of the heart
    - Natrum mur. 6x
    - Calc.sulph. 6x
    - Silicea 6x

12. Regurgitation or Reflux of food
 Kali.phos. 6x
 Natrum sulph. 6x
 Calc.sulph. 6x
13. Vertigo with dyspepsia
 Natrum sulph. 6x
 Kali.sulph. 6x
 Calc.sulph. 6x

DYSPHAGIA (Difficulty in swallowing) (See GERD also)
 Natrum sulph. 6x
 Kali.sulph. 6x
 Calc.sulph. 6x

DYSPNOEA (Breathlessness)
1. Aggravation by lying down
 Kali.sulph. 6x
 Calc.sulph. 6x
 Silicea 6x
2. Aggravation by sitting up
 Calc.phos. 6x
 Calc.flor. 6x
 Silicea 6x
3. Aggravation by walking
 Kali.mur. 6x
 Calc.sulph. 6x
 Calc.flor. 6x
4. Aggravation from working
 Kali.mur. 6x
 Kali.sulph. 6x
 Calc.sulph. 6x
5. Relief from expectoration
 Natrum sulph. 6x
 Calc.sulph. 6x
 Silicea 6x

6. Relief from sitting up
      Kali.phos. 6x
      Kali.sulph. 6x
      Calc.sulph. 6x

DYSPNOEA-Bronchial
1. Gasping breathing
      Natrum sulph. 6x
      Calc.sulph. 6x
      Silicea 6x
2. Rattling breathing
      Kali.phos. 6x
      Natrum sulph. 6x
      Calc.sulph. 6x
3. Suffocative breathing, difficult breathing
      Natrum sulph. 6x
      Kali.sulph. 6x
      Calc.sulph. 6x

DYSPONEA-Cardiac,(cardiac asthma due to heart disease)
      Natrum sulph. 6x
      Kali.sulph. 6x
      Silicea 6x

DYSURIA (Painful, difficult urination)
1. General formula
      Natrum sulph. 6x
      Kali.sulph. 6x
      Calc.sulph. 6x
2. Pregnancy and after (Painful urination)
      Natrum sulph. 6x
      Calc.sulph. 6x
      Silicea 6x
3. Newly married women: (Honey-moon cystitis)
      Kali.sulph. 6x
      Calc.sulph. 6x
      Silicea 6x

4. With prostate disease (Painful urination)
   Natrum mur. 6x
   Kali.mur. 6x
   Calc.sulph. 6x
5. With uterine diseases (Painful urination)
   Kali.sulph. 6x
   Calc.sulph. 6x
   Calc.flor. 6x
6. Feeble stream of urine (Painful urination)
   Natrum sulph. 6x
   Kali.sulph. 6x
   Calc.sulph. 6x

E

EAR DISEASES See External auditory canal, Deafness, Earache, Otitis (inflammation of ear), Otalgia (pain in ear), Otorrhea).

EAR DISCHARGE (See Otorrhea)
EAR WAX-deficient

Natrum sulph.	6x
Calc.sulph.	6x
Silicea	6x

EARACHE, Otalgia (Pain in ear)
    Pulsating, throbbing pain

Natrum sulph.	6x
Kali.sulph.	6x
Calc.sulph.	6x

EAR, as if obstructed

Kali.mur.	6x
Calc.sulph.	6x
Calc.flor.	6x

EBOLA VIRUS DISEASE (Ebola haemorrhagic fever)

Natrum sulph.	30x
Kali.sulph.	6x
Calc.sulph.	6x

Dose: 2 hourly for 3-5 days and then 4 hourly.
Prevention: once daily during the epidemic.

ECCHYMOSIS (Red, pink or bluish spots below skin due to subcutaneous bleeding)

Natrum mur.	6x
Natrum sulph.	6x
Calc.sulph.	6x

ECLAMPSIA (Hypertension, albuminuria and fits during pregnancy)

Kali.sulph.	12x
Kali.mur.	12x
Natrum mur.	12x

Dose: Give half hourly till the improvement occurs.

ECTROPION (See Eyes)

ECZEMA

1. Dry eczema with itching
   - Natrum mur. 6x
   - Kali.mur. 6x
   - Calc.sulph. 6x
2. Wet eczema (eczema with discharge)
   - Calc.phos. 6x
   - Ferrum phos 6x
   - Calc.sulph. 6x

ELECTRIC SHOCK

- Natrum sulph. 6x
- Kali.sulph. 6x
- Calc.sulph. 6x

Dose: Give after every half hour till the improvement occurs.

ELEPHANTIASIS (a disease of lymphatic system, caused by a mosquito transmitted parasite, named filaria).
- Kali.sulph. 6x
- Calc.sulph. 6x
- Silicea 200x

EMISSIONS (nocturnal pollutions; sexual debility)

1. General formula
   - Kali.phos. 6x
   - Natrum mur. 6x
   - Kali.mur. 6x
2. With brain-fag, weak legs and backache
   - Natrum mur. 6x
   - Kali.mur. 6x
   - Calc.sulph. 6x
3. Emissions-diurnal (day time), by straining at stool
   - Kali.phos. 6x
   - Kali.mur. 6x
   - Calc.sulph. 6x

4. Emissions-premature (premature ejaculation)

	Natrum sulph.	6x
	Kali.sulph.	6x
	Calc.sulph.	6x

5. Emissions-with weak erections

	Kali.sulph.	6x
	Calc.sulph.	6x
	Kali.mur.	6x

6. Emissions-with irritability, despondency, depression

	Calc.sulph.	6x
	Kali.sulph.	6x
	Kali.mur.	6x

(See Sexual disorders also)

EMPHYSEMA (See Lungs)

EMPYEMA (See Pleurisy, Pleuritis)

ENCEPHALITIS LETHARGICA (Sleeping sickness)

	Kali.phos.	6x
	Kali.sulph.	6x
	Calc.sulph.	6x

ENCOPARESIS (A psychological and neuro-developmental disorder of childhood in which repeated passage, usually involuntary, of stools occurs).

	Natrum sulph.	6x
	Kali.sulph.	6x
	Calc.sulph.	6x

ENDOCARDITIS (See Heart)

ENDOMETRIOSIS (presence of endometrial tissue outside the uterus, causing pain and menstrual problems).

	Natrum mur.	6x
	Calc.sulph.	6x
	Silicea	6x

ENDOCERVICITIS	See Uterus
ENDOMETRITIS	See Uterus
ENTERALGIA	See Colic

ENTERIC DISEASES FROM ANIMALS

Kali.sulph.	6x
Calc.sulph.	6x
Calc.flor.	6x
Silicea	6x

ENTERITIS (See Diarrhea)
ENTROPION (See Eyes)
ENURESIS (Involuntary urination)
1. General remedy for involuntary urination

Natrum sulph.	6x
Kali.mur.	6x
Kali.sulph.	6x

2. Diurnal (day time-enuresis

Natrum sulph.	6x
Kali.sulph.	6x
Calc.sulph.	6x

3. Nocturnal (during night in sleep)-enuresis

Kali.phos.	6x
Natrum mur.	6x
Calc.sulph.	6x

4. Weak or paretic sphincter of bladder-enuresis

Kali.phos.	6x
Calc.sulph.	6x
Silicea	6x

(See Urine also)

ENNVIRONMENTAL EXPOSURE - BAD EFFECTS

Kali.sulph.	6x
Natrum sulph.	6x
Calc.sulph.	6x

EOSINOPHILIA

Natrum sulph.	6x
Kali.sulph.	6x
Calc.sulph.	6x

EPIDIDYMITIS (See Testes)

EPILEPSY

1. Grand Mal epilepsy
    - Kali.sulph.   6x
    - Calc.sulph.   6x
    - Silicea   6x
2. Petit mal epilepsy
    - Kali.phos.   6x
    - Natrum mur.   6x
    - Kali sulph.   6x
3. From fright, emotional causes
    - Kali.phos.   6x
    - Natrum sulph.   6x
    - Calc.sulph.   6x
4. From fever (Febrile fits)
    - Natrum sulph.   6x
    - Kali.sulph.   6x
    - Calc.sulph.   6x
5. From head injury
    - Natrum mur.   6x
    - Kali.sulph.   6x
    - Calc.sulph.   6x
6. From worms
    - Kali.mur.   6x
    - Calc.sulph.   6x
    - Silicea   6x
7. In children
    - Kali.phos.   6x
    - Natrum sulph.   6x
    - Calc.sulph.   6x
8. Preceded by sudden cry
    - Kali.phos.   6x
    - Kali.sulph.   6x
    - Calc.sulph.   6x
9. Status epilepticus (severe attack of epilepsy)
    - Kali.phos.   6x
    - Natrum sulph.   6x
    - Kali sulph.   6x

EPIPHORA (excessive flow of water from one or both eyes).
- Nat.phos. 6x
- Natrum sulph. 6x
- Calc.sulph. 6x

EPISTAXIS (See Nose)

EPITHELIOMA (Tumor or abnormal growth of epithelium).
- Kali.phos. 6x
- Natrum mur. 6x
- Kali.mur. 6x

ERECTILE DYSFUNCTION (See Impotence, Sex disorders)
- Kali.phos. 6x
- Natrum sulph. 6x
- Calc.sulph. 6x

EROTOMANIA (See Mania)

ERUCTATIONS (See Dyspepsia)

ERYSIPELAS (Infection with fiery red rash of upper layers of skin caused by a bacterium, srtreprococccus pyogenes.)
- Kali.phos. 6x
- Kali sulph. 6x
- Calc.sulph. 6x

Constitutional tendency-of erysipelas
- Kali.mur. 6x
- Kali.sulph. 6x
- Calc.sulph. 6x

ERYTHEMA (Mild to life threatening skin rash caused by a disease, infection or drugs.)

1. Inertrigo (Chaffing)
   - Kali.sulph. 6x
   - Calc.sulph. 6x
   - Silicea 6x

2. Erythem multiforme
   - Kali.sulph. 6x
   - Calc.sulph. 6x
   - Silicea 6x

3. Erythema Simplex

  Kali.sulph. 6x
  Calc.flor. 6x
  Silicea 6x

ESCHERICHIA COLI INFECTION (E. coli)

  Kali.sulph. 6x
  Calc.sulph. 6x
  Calc.flor. 6x
  Silicea 6x

EUSTACHIAN DEAFNESS (See Deafness)

EUTHYROID SICK SYNDROME

  Ferrum phos 6x
  Natrum sulph. 6x
  Calc.sulph. 6x

EXHAUSTION (See Weakness)

EXOPHTHALMIC GOITRE (See Goitre)

EXOSTOSIS (See Bones)

EXTERNAL AUDITORY CANAL

1. Boils, pimples-in external auditory canal

  Kali.mur. 6x
  Calc.sulph. 6x
  Silicea 6x

2. Digging and scratching into auditory canal

  Natrum mur. 6x
  Kali.mur. 6x
  Calc.sulph. 6x

3. Ear wax, deficiency

  Natrum sulph. 6x
  Calc.sulph. 6x
  Silicea 6x

4. Fungal infectionof ear

  Natrum sulph. 6x
  Kali.mur. 6x
  Calc.sulph. 6x

5. Inflammation and pain in auditory canal

Kali.sulph.	6x
Calc.sulph.	6x
Silicea	6x

6. Itching in auditory canal

Natrum mur.	6x
Kali.mur.	6x
Calc.sulph.	6x

7. Sensation, as if heat emanated from auditory canal

Natrum sulph.	6x
Kali.sulph.	6x
Calc.sulph.	6x

8. Sensation, as if obstructed, auditory canal or ear

Kali.mur.	6x
Calc.sulph.	6x
Silicea	6x

EYE DISEASES

1. Acute haemorrhagic conjunctivitis

Natrum sulph.	6x
Kali.sulph.	6x
Calc.sulph.	6x

2. Agglutination of eyelids

Kali.sulph.	6x
Calc.sulph.	6x
Silicea	6x

3. Catarat (See Cataract)

4. Drooping (ptosis or paralysis of upper eylelids)

Kali.phos.	6x
Kali.mur.	6x
Calc.flor.	6x

5. Dryness of eyes

Calc.phos.	6x
Natrum mur.	6x
Kali.mur.	6x

6. Ectropion (Outward turning of eyelids and eyelashes)
   - Kali.phos. 6x
   - Kali.sulph. 6x
   - Calc.sulph. 6x
7. Entropion (inward turning of eyelids and eyelashes)
   - Kali.phos. 6x
   - Kali.mur. 6x
   - Silicea 6x
8. Epiphora (See Epiphora)
9. Glaucoma
   - Natrum sulph. 6x
   - Kali.sulph. 6x
   - Calc.sulph. 6x
10. Ophthlmia (See Eyes)
11. Keratoconus
    - Kali.phos. 6x
    - Natrum sulph. 6x
    - Kali sulph. 6x
12. Optic nerve (See Optic)
13. Optical or vision disorders (See Optical)
14. Pupils, contracted (miosis)
    - Calc.sulph. 6x
    - Calc.flor. 6x
    - Silicea 6x
15. Dilated pupils (mydriasis)
    - Kali.phos. 6x
    - Natrum sulph. 6x
    - Calc.sulph. 6x
16. Retina (See Retina)
17. Scleritis (inflammation of scleral tissue of eye)
    - Calc.phos. 6x
    - Natrum sulph. 6x
    - Calc.sulph. 6x

EYELIDS - GROWTHS
1. Chalazion, trasal tumors
   - Kali.mur. 6x
   - Calc.sulph. 6x
   - Silicea 6x
2. Cysts, sebaceous
   - Natrum sulph. 6x
   - Kali.sulph. 6x
   - Calc.sulph. 6x
3. Granular lids (Trachoma)
   - Kali.phos. 6x
   - Natrum sulph. 6x
   - Calc.sulph. 6x
4. Pterygium (See Pterygium)
   - Natrum sulph. 6x
   - Kali.sulph. 6x
   - Calc.flor. 6x
5. Styes (Hordeolum)(inflammation of gland or follicle in eyelid)
   - Natrum sulph. 6x
   - Kali.sulph. 6x
   - Calc.sulph. 6x
6. Inflammation of eye lid margin (Blepharitis)
   a. Acute blepharitis
   - Natrum sulph. 6x
   - Kali.sulph. 6x
   - Calc.sulph. 6x
   b. Chronic blepharitis
   - Calc.sulph. 6x
   - Calc.flor. 6x
   - Silicea 6x

EYES - OPTICAL ILLUSIONS
1. Flashes, flames, stars
   - Kali.phos. 6x
   - Natrum sulph. 6x
   - Kali sulph. 6x

2. Halo around light
                                Kali.phos.   6x
                                Natrum sulph.   6x
                                Silicea   6x
3. Spots, floaters (muscae volitantes)
                                Kali.phos.   6x
                                Kali.mur.   6x
                                Calc.sulph.   6x

F

FACE - COMPLEXION, to make it fair
- Natrum mur. 6x
- Ferrum phos 6x
- Calc.sulph. 6x

External application: Calc. flor-3x cream, twice daily.

FACE - APPEARANCE
1. Anaemic face
   - Ferrum phos 6x
   - Natrum sulph. 6x
   - Calc.sulph. 6x
2. Anxious looking, suffering expression of face
   - Mag.phos. 6x
   - Kali.mur. 6x
   - Silicea 6x
3. Bloated, puffiness, around eyes
   - Kali.sulph. 6x
   - Calc.sulph. 6x
   - Silicea 6x
4. Bloated, swollen, lower eyelids
   - Calc.phos. 6x
   - Natrum sulph. 6x
   - Calc.sulph. 6x
5. Bloated, puffy face
   - Natrum sulph. 6x
   - Kali.sulph. 6x
   - Calc.sulph. 6x
6. Blue, livid (cyanosis)-face
   - Natrum sulph. 6x
   - Kali.sulph. 6x
   - Calc.sulph. 6x
7. Blue rings, around eyes
   - Natrum mur. 6x
   - Kali.mur. 6x
   - Calc.sulph. 6x

8. Blushing-face
    Kali.sulph. 6x
    Calc.sulph. 6x
    Silicea 6x
9. Brown spots, on face
    Kali.phos. 6x
    Natrum mur. 6x
    Calc.sulph. 6x
10. Bronzed-face
    Natrum sulph. 6x
    Kali.sulph. 6x
    Calc.sulph. 6x
11. Distorted face
    Kali.phos. 6x
    Natrum sulph. 6x
    Calc.sulph. 6x
12. Drowsy, stupid face
    Kali.sulph. 6x
    Calc.sulph. 6x
    Silicea 6x
13. Earthy, unwashed, dirty looking face
    Natrum sulph. 6x
    Kali.sulph. 6x
    Calc.sulph. 6x
14. Hippocratic (sickly, sunken, deathly cold) face
    Calc.phos. 6x
    Kali.phos. 6x
    Natrum sulph. 6x
15. Jaundiced, yellow face
    Natrum sulph. 6x
    Kali.sulph. 6x
    Calc.sulph. 6x
16. Mask-like, expressionless face
    Kali.phos. 6x
    Kali.mur. 6x
    Silicea 6x

17. Oily, shiny face
          Natrum mur. 6x
          Kali.sulph. 6x
          Calc.sulph. 6x
18. Pale face
          Kali.mur. 6x
          Kali.sulph. 6x
          Calc.sulph. 6x
19. Red face
          Natrum sulph. 6x
          Calc.sulph. 6x
          Silicea 6x
20. Sweating, on face
          Kali.phos. 6x
          Kali.mur. 6x
          Calc.sulph. 6x
21. Swelling, of face
          Calc.phos. 6x
          Natrum sulph. 6x
          Calc.sulph. 6x
22. Wrinkled, old-looking face
          Kali.phos. 6x
          Kali.mur. 6x
          Calc.sulph. 6x

FACE - BONES
1. Caries (exostosis, inflammation)
          Kali sulph. 6x
          Calc.sulph. 6x
          Calc.flor. 6x
2. Coldness, feeling in bones of face
          Calc.phos. 6x
          Kali.sulph. 6x
          Natrum mur. 6x
3. Pain in bones of face
          Calc.sulph. 6x
          Kali sulph. 6x
          Silicea 6x

FACE - CHEEKS

1. Bites cheeks, when chewing, talking
   - Kali.phos. 6x
   - Natrum mur. 6x
   - Calc.sulph. 6x
2. Burning, hot cheeks
   - Ferrum phos 6x
   - Natrum sulph. 6x
   - Calc.sulph. 6x
3. Eruptions on cheeks
   - Natrum sulph. 6x
   - Kali.sulph. 6x
   - Calc.sulph. 6x
4. Formication, numb, tingling, crawling-sensation
   - Calc.phos. 6x
   - Kali.phos. 6x
   - Natrum sulph. 6x
5. Redness of cheeks
   - Ferrum phos 6x
   - Natrum sulph. 6x
   - Kali sulph. 6x
6. Yellow saddle around nose (lupus)
   - Kali.phos. 6x
   - Natrum sulph. 6x
   - Calc.sulph. 6x

FACE - Eruptions on chin
- Natrum mur. 6x
- Kali.mur. 6x
- Calc.sulph. 6x

FACE - ERUPTIONS

1. Acne (See Acne)

2. Chilblains (red or black spots due to cold)
   - Kali.phos. 6x
   - Natrum mur. 6x
   - Calc.sulph. 6x

3. Comedones
balckheads (open comedones) or *whiteheads (closed comedones)*

Kali.sulph.	6x
Calc.sulph.	6x
Silicea	6x

4. Eczema, face

Natrum mur.	6x
Kali.mur.	6x
Calc.sulph.	6x

5. Erysipelas (see erysipelas also)

Kali.phos.	6x
Kali sulph.	6x
Calc.sulph.	6x

6. Frackles (Lentigo)

Ferrum phos	6x
Kali.mur.	6x
Calc.sulph.	6x

7. Frost-bite-face

Kali.mur.	6x
Calc.sulph.	6x
Silicea	6x

8. Herpes simplex

Natrum sulph.	6x
Kali.sulph.	6x
Calc.sulph.	6x

9. Pustules of face

Natrum mur.	6x
Natrum sulph.	6x
Kali.mur.	6x

10. Spots, copper colored, on face

Kali.phos.	6x
Natrum sulph.	6x
Calc.sulph.	6x

11. Whiskers, eruptions, falling out, itching

Kali.sulph.	6x
Calc.sulph.	6x
Silicea	6x

FACE WASHING - ameliorates

Kali.mur.	6x
Kali.sulph.	6x
Calc.sulph.	6x

FACE- PROSOPALGIA (See trigeminal neuralgia)

FAINTING (See Syncope also)

Kali.phos.	6x
Natrum sulph.	6x
Calc.sulph.	6x

FALLOPIAN TUBES
1. General formula for fallopian tubes, diseases

Kali.phos.	6x
Calc.sulph.	6x
Silicea	6x

2. Blocked fallopian tubes

Kali.phos.	6x
Calc.sulph.	6x
Calc.flor.	6x

3. Inflammation of fallopian tubes (Salpingitis)

Kali.sulph.	6x
Calc.sulph.	6x
Calc.flor.	6x

FARMER'S LUNG (Lungs inflammation due to inhalation of biological dusts)

Natrum sulph.	6x
Kali.sulph.	6x
Calc.sulph.	6x

FATIGUE

Natrum sulph.	6x
Kali.mur.	6x
Calc.sulph.	6x

FATTY LIVER

1. Alcoholic fatty liver
   - Kali.mur. 6x
   - Kali.sulph. 6x
   - Calc.sulph. 6x
2. Non-alcoholic fatty liver
   - Calc.sulph. 6x
   - Calc.flor. 6x
   - Silicea 6x
3. Fatty liver with obesity and PCOD
   - Kali.phos. 6x
   - Kali.sulph. 6x
   - Calc.flor. 6x
4. Fatty liver with gall stones
   - Natrum sulph. 6x
   - Kali sulph. 6x
   - Calc.sulph. 6x

FEARS

1. Being carried or raised- in children
   - Kali.sulph. 6x
   - Calc.sulph. 6x
   - Silicea 6x
2. Claustrophobia (fear of confined or close spaces)
   - Kali.phos. 6x
   - Kali.sulph. 6x
   - Calc.sulph. 6x
3. Crossing streets, crowds, excitement
   - Calc.sulph. 6x
   - Calc.flor. 6x
   - Silicea 6x
4. Death, fatal diseases, impending evils
   - Kali.sulph. 6x
   - Calc.sulph. 6x
   - Silicea 6x
5. People (Anthropophobia)
   - Kali.phos. 6x
   - Natrum mur. 6x
   - Kali.mur. 6x

6. Stage fright

Kali.phos.	6x
Natrum sulph.	6x
Kali sulph.	6x

7. Water fear (Hydrophobia)

Kali.phos.	6x
Kali.mur.	6x
Calc.sulph.	6x

FEBRILE FITS (See Epilepsy)

FECAL INCONTINENCE (Loss of control of stool)

Kali.phos.	30x
Natrum sulph.	6x
Calc.sulph.	6x

FELON (Abscess near finger nail or toe nail)

Kali.sulph.	6x
Calc.sulph.	6x
Silicea	6x

FEVER

Sponging with normal tap water is very effective.
General formula for fevers

Calc.sulph.	6x
Ferrum phos	6x
Natrum sulph.	6x
Natrum mur.	6x

FEVER - TYPES

1. Dengue fever   (See dengue fever)
2. Ebola fever   (See ebola fever)
3. Malaria   (See malaria)
4. Rheumatic fever   (See rheumatic fever)
5. Tonsillitis   (See tonsillitis)
6. Typhoid fever   (See typhoid fever)
7. Viral infections (See Common cold, Flu, Dengue fever, Ebola virus, Zika virus and other symptoms).

FEVER - CONCOMITANTS

1. With bronchitis
   - Ferrum phos   6x
   - Natrum sulph.   6x
   - Kali.sulph.   6x
   - Calc.sulph.   6x

2. With colicky pain in abdomen and foul-smelling stool
   - Natrum sulph.   6x
   - Kali.sulph.   6x
   - Silicea   6x

3. With eruptions like Measles, Chicken-Pox
   - Natrum mur.   6x
   - Natrum sulph.   6x
   - Calc.sulph.   6x

4. With tonsillitis
   - Calc.phos.   6x
   - Kali.phos.   6x
   - Calc.sulph.   6x

5. With influenza
   - Natrum mur.   6x
   - Kali.mur.   6x
   - Calc.sulph.   6x

6. Malaria, with shaking chill
   - Natrum sulph.   6x
   - Kali.sulph.   6x
   - Calc.sulph.   6x

7. Septic fever
   - Kali.phos.   6x
   - Natrum sulph.   6x
   - Calc.sulph.   6x

8. Fever, due to vaccination
   - Natrum sulph.   6x
   - Kali.sulph.   6x
   - Silicea   6x

FIBROID TUMORS-uterus

Kali.sulph. 6x
Calc.sulph. 6x
Calc.flor. 6x

(See Tumors also)
FIBROMYALGIA (Pain in muscles and bones alongwith weakness, memory, sleep and mood problems).

Natrum sulph. 6x
Kali.sulph. 6x
Calc.sulph. 6x

FIBROSIS LUNGS

Natrum sulph. 6x
Calc.sulph.
Silicea

FINGERS
1. Cracks in skin

   Natrum mur. 6x
   Kali.mur. 6x
   Calc.sulph. 6x

2. Cracking sound in finger joints

   Natrum sulph. 6x
   Kali.mur. 6x
   Calc.sulph. 6x

3. Finger joints-pain, swelling, stiffness

   Ferrum phos 6x
   Mag.phos. 6x
   Natrum sulph. 6x

4. Finger joints-deformed

   Natrum mur. 6x
   Kali.mur. 6x
   Calc.flor. 6x

5. habit of putting fingers into mouth - (in children)

   Kali.sulph. 6x
   Calc.sulph. 6x
   Silicea 6x

6. habit putting fingers into mouth (in adults)
 - Kali.phos 6x
 - Natrum sulph. 6x
 - Natrum mur. 6x

7. Mouth, putting fingers into - (autistic children)
 - Calc.suph. 6x
 - Kali.sulph. 6x
 - Natrum sulph. 6x

8. Nodes in finger joints
 - Calc.phos. 6x
 - Natrum sulph. 6x
 - Calc.flor. 6x

FISTULA

1. Anus (Fistula in ano)
 - Kali.phos. 6x
 - Natrum sulph. 6x
 - Kali.sulph. 6x
 - Calc.sulph. 6x

2. Dental fistula (See Teeth)

FITS, CONVULSIONS (See Epilepsy)

FLU, INFLUENZAVIRAL RESPIRATORY INFECTIONS
(See flu, influenza, coryza, cough, fever, pharyngitis, bronchitis, viral diseases, severe acute respiratory syndrome, asphyxia, cyanosis, avian influenza, septicemia, bird flu, cyanosis, multiple organ dysfunction syndrome, bronchospam, cough, pneumonia, swine flu, coma, blood clotting, clotting of blood and oxygen-low saturation and other relevant symptoms).

Following formulas can be used in any disease according to the symptoms-similarity.

1. General formula
 - Natrum mur. 6x
 - Kali.sulph. 6x
 - Calc.sulph. 6x
 - Calc.flor. 6x
 - Silicea 6x

2. Cough, fever, dyspnea, blood clotting, shock, lung fibrosis, low oxygen saturation in blood-leading to shock and even death.
   Kali.sulph. 6x
   Calc.sulph. 6x
   Silicea 6x
3. Blue lips and tongue (cyanosis), with flu
   Kali.phos. 6x
   Mag.phos. 6x
   Nat.phos. 6x
4. Dry cough
   Natrum mur. 6x
   Natrum sulph. 6x
   Kali sulph. 6x
5. Difficulty in breathing, with
   Natrum mur. 6x
   Natrum sulph. 6x
   Calc.sulph. 6x
6. Chronic cough
   Natrum sulph. 6x
   Kali.sulph. 6x
   Calc.sulph. 6x
7. Fever, with
   Natrum sulph. 6x
   Kali.mur. 6x
   Calc.sulph. 6x
8. Fever and chills, with
   Kali.mur. 6x
   Kali.sulph. 6x
   Calc.sulph. 6x
9. Hoarse, hollow, metallic cough
   Natrum sulph. 6x
   Kali.sulph. 6x
   Calc.sulph. 6x

10. Low oxygen saturation in blood, with
　　　　　　　　　　　　Kali.sulph.　6x
　　　　　　　　　　　　Calc.sulph.　6x
　　　　　　　　　　　　Silicea　　　6x
11. Septicemia, with
　　　　　　　　　　　　Calc.phos.　6x
　　　　　　　　　　　　Kali.mur.　　6x
　　　　　　　　　　　　Calc.sulph.　6x
　　　　　　　　　　　　Silicea　　　6x
12. Shock and collapse, with
　　　　　　　　　　　　Kali.sulph.　6x
　　　　　　　　　　　　Calc.sulph.　6x
　　　　　　　　　　　　Calc.flor.　 6x
　　　　　　　　　　　　Silicea　　　6x
13. Weakness, extreme, with
　　　　　　　　　　　　Kali.sulph.　6x
　　　　　　　　　　　　Calc.sulph.　6x
　　　　　　　　　　　　Calc.flor.　 6x
　　　　　　　　　　　　Silicea　　　6x
　　　　(See common cold also)

FLU - PREVENTION - for prevention of all types of flu and other viral infections.
(Contacts of patients and health care/laboratory workers/ all other staff of hospitals).
　　　　　　　　　　　　Kali.phos.　6x
　　　　　　　　　　　　Kali.sulph.　6x
　　　　　　　　　　　　Calc.sulph.　6x
Dose: once daily for one month and on alternate days to children (5-12 years age), for one month.
Prevention in Children below 4 years age: Once daily for one month.
(See the other symtoms of viral diseases in various parts of this book, and treat accordingly).

FLATULENCE (Gas in stomach and intestines)

Natrum sulph.	6x
Calc.sulph.	6x
Silicea	6x

(See Dyspepsia, Indigestion also)

FOLLICULITIS (Inflammation or infection of a hair follicle).

Natrum sulph.	6x
Kali.sulph.	6x
Calc.sulph.	6x

FOOD ALLERGIES (See Allergies)

FOOD POISONING

Kali.phos.	6x
Kali.mur.	6x
Calc.sulph.	6x

Dose: repeat after every 15 minutes, till improvent starts.

FOODS - THAT DISAGREE

1. General formula for food problems

Natrum mur.	6x
Natrum sulph.	6x
Kali.mur.	6x

2. Bread disagrees

Kali.phos.	6x
Natrum mur.	6x
Calc.sulph.	6x

3. Butter disagrees

Natrum mur.	6x
Kali.mur.	6x
Calc.flor.	6x

4. Cabbage diagrees

Natrum mur.	6x
Kali.mur.	6x
Calc.sulph.	6x

5. Cheese disagrees

Natrum mur.	6x
Natrum sulph.	6x
Kali.mur.	6x

6. Egg and egg products disagree
                                  Kali.phos.   6x
                                  Natrum sulph.   6x
                                  Calc.sulph.   6x

7. Fats disagree
                                  Natrum sulph.   6x
                                  Kali.mur.   6x
                                  Calc.sulph.   6x

8. Food of any kind, disagree
                                  Natrum mur.   6x
                                  Kali.sulph.   6x
                                  Calc.sulph.   6x

9. Fruits disagree
                                  Kali.mur.   6x
                                  Calc.sulph.   6x
                                  Calc.flor.   6x

10. Milk disagrees
                                  Natrum sulph.   6x
                                  Kali.sulph.   6x
                                  Calc.sulph.   6x

11. Pastry, cake, bakery items, disagree
                                  Kali.mur.   6x
                                  Calc.sulph.   6x
                                  Calc.flor.   6x

12. Potatoes disagree
                                  Calc.sulph.   6x
                                  Calc.flor.   6x
                                  Silicea   6x

13. Spicy foods, disagree
                                  Natrum mur.   6x
                                  Calc.sulph.   6x
                                  Calc.flor.   6x

14. Sour foods, disagree
                                  Calc.sulph.   6x
                                  Calc.flor.   6x
                                  Silicea   6x

15. Sweets, disagree

    Kali.sulph. 6x
    Calc.sulph. 6x
    Calc.flor. 6x

FOOT DISEASES

1. Arthritis of joints of feet

    Ferrum phos 6x
    Kali.sulph. 6x
    Calc.sulph. 6x

2. Athlete's foot (Fungal inection called tinea pedis which occurs in the skin, in between the toes)

    Mag.phos. 6x
    Nat.phos. 6x
    Natrum sulph. 6x

3. Deformed joints of feet

    Kali.phos. 6x
    Mag.phos. 6x
    Calc.flor. 6x

4. Foot drop (Inability to lift the front part of foot)

    Natrum sulph. 6x
    Kali.mur. 6x
    Calc.sulph. 6x

5. Numbness of toes

    Kali.phos. 6x
    Natrum sulph. 6x
    Calc.sulph. 6x

6. Oedema of feet

    Natrum sulph. 6x
    Kali.mur. 6x
    Calc.sulph. 6x

7. Pain in big toe

    Calc.phos. 6x
    Ferrum phos 6x
    Natrum sulph. 6x

8. Pain in heel
 - Kali.sulph. 6x
 - Calc.sulph. 6x
 - Silicea 6x

9. Pain in soles, plantar fasciitis
 - Kali.phos. 6x
 - Natrum sulph. 6x
 - Calc.sulph. 6x

10. Pain in toes
 - Kali.phos. 6x
 - Natrum mur. 6x
 - Calc.sulph. 6x

11. Sweating in foot, excessive and bad smelling
 (See Sweating)

FOREARM

1. Pain in forearm
 - Natrum sulph. 6x
 - Kali.sulph. 6x
 - Calc.sulph. 6x

2. Wasting of muscles of forearm
 - Kali.phos. 6x
 - Kali.sulph. 6x
 - Calc.sulph. 6x

3. Weakness of forearm or as if paralyzed
 - Kali.phos. 6x
 - Natrum sulph. 6x
 - Calc.sulph. 6x

FRACTURES

- Natrum mur. 6x
- Kali.sulph. 6x
- Calc.sulph. 6x

(See Bones also)

FRECKLES (lentigo)

- Ferrum phos 6x
- Kali.mur. 6x
- Calc.sulph. 6x

(See Face also)

FRIGIDITY (See Sex desire,decreasesd, in females)
FROST BITE

          Kali.phos.   6x
          Natrum mur.   6x
          Calc.sulph.   6x

FROZEN SHOULDER (Adhesive capsulitis) (See Shoulder)
FUNGAL INFECTIONS
  General formula

          Ferrum phos   6x
          Kali.mur.   6x
          Calc.sulph.   6x

(See Athelete's foot, Candidiasis, Pityriasis, Ringworm, Sinusitis-fungal, Onychomycosis, External auditory canal, Tinea capitis,Tinea versicolor)

FURUNCLE (Infection of a hair follicle)

          Calc.sulph.   6x
          Kali.sulph.   6x
          Natrum sulph.   6x

Recurrent boils or furuncles

          Kali.sulph.   6x
          Calc.sulph.   6x
          Silicea   6x

G

GAIT DISORDERS
1. Ataxic gait (See Locomotor Ataxia also)
   - Kali.phos. 6x
   - Natrum mur. 6x
   - Calc.sulph. 6x
2. Child-slow to learn walking
   - Kali.phos. 6x
   - Calc.sulph. 6x
   - Natrum sulph. 6x
3. Child - walks on toes
   - Kali.phos. 6x
   - Calc.sulph. 6x
   - Natrum sulph. 6x
4. Drags feet, when walking
   - Kali.sulph. 6x
   - Calc.sulph. 6x
   - Calc.flor. 6x
5. Sluggish, Slow gait
   - Kali.phos. 6x
   - Kali.mur. 6x
   - Calc.sulph. 6x
6. Staggering, unsteady gait
   - Kali.phos. 6x
   - Natrum mur. 6x
   - Kali.mur. 6x
7. Stumbles easily, when walking
   - Kali.phos. 6x
   - Natrum sulph. 6x
   - Kali sulph. 6x

GALACTORRHOEA (Excessive milk secretion)
- Kali.sulph. 6x
- Calc.sulph. 6x
- Calc.flor. 6x

(See Breasts also)

GALL-STONES
1. Colic and inflammation of gall bladder
   - Natrum mur. 6x
   - Kali.mur. 6x
   - Calc.sulph. 6x
2. Cholilithiasis (Gall stones) - to dissolve
   - Kali.phos. 6x
   - Natrum sulph. 6x
   - Calc.sulph. 6x

(See Colic also)

GANGLION, on back of wrist and other places
- Kali.sulph. 6x
- Calc.sulph. 6x
- Silicea 6x

GANGRENE (Death of body tissue due to absence of blood circulation, bacterial infection or trauma)
1. General formula
   - Kali.sulph. 6x
   - Calc.sulph. 6x
   - Calc.flor. 6x
   - Silicea 6x
2. Senile gangrene (gangrene in old age)
   - Kali.sulph. 6x
   - Calc.sulph. 6x
   - Silicea 6x
3. Traumatic gangrene (due to injury)
   - Kali.sulph. 6x
   - Calc.sulph. 6x
   - Calc.flor. 6x
   - Silicea 6x

GAS FUMES - ill effects of (carbon monoxide, coal gas, sewer gas and all other poisonous gases)
- Kali.phos. 6x
- Natrum sulph. 6x
- Calc.sulph. 6x

Repeat one dose after every 5 minutes, till the improvemet.

GASTRIC PAIN
1. Burning in stomach, as from ulcer
   - Nat.phos. 6x
   - Natrum sulph. 6x
   - Kali sulph. 6x
2. Crampy, colicky gastric pain
   - Calc.phos. 6x
   - Mag.phos. 6x
   - Calc.sulph. 6x
3. Cutting, paroxysmal, spasmodic gastric pain
   - Natrum sulph. 6x
   - Kali.sulph. 6x
   - Calc.sulph. 6x
4. Epigastric (pit of stomach), pain
   - Kali.sulph. 6x
   - Calc.sulph. 6x
   - Silicea 6x
5. Gnawing, hungry-like, gastric pain
   - Kali.sulph. 6x
   - Calc.sulph. 6x
   - Silicea 6x

GASTRIC PAIN - **Aggravation of gastric pain**
1. Empty stomach, aggravates pain
   - Silicea 6x
   - Calc.flor. 6x
   - Calc.sulph. 6x
2. From eating food
   - Silicea 6x
   - Calc.sulph. 6x
   - Calc.flor. 6x

GASTRIC PAIN - **Amelioration of gastric pain**
1. From bending backward, standing erect
   - Kali.mur. 6x
   - Kali.sulph. 6x
   - Calc.sulph. 6x

2. From eating, pain is relieved
   - Kali.sulph. 6x
   - Calc.sulph. 6x
   - Silicea 6x
3. From pressure
   - Natrum sulph. 6x
   - Kali.sulph. 6x
   - Calc.sulph. 6x

GASTRITIS (Inflammation of mucosa of stomach)
1. Acute gastriris
   - Ferrum phos 6x
   - Mag.phos. 6x
   - Natrum sulph. 6x
2. Acute gastritis, from alcohol abuse
   - Natrum mur. 6x
   - Natrum sulph. 6x
   - Calc.sulph. 6x
3. Acute gastritis, with intestinal involvement
   - Calc.phos. 6x
   - Natrum mur. 6x
   - Kali.mur. 6x
4. Chronic gastritis (chronic inflammation of stomach)
   - Kali.phos. 6x
   - Natrum mur. 6x
   - Silicea 6x

GATSRO-ENTERITIS
   - Kali.phos. 6x
   - Natrum sulph. 6x
   - Calc.sulph. 6x

GENITOURINARY SYSTEM (See Sexual disorders, Testes, Semen, Sperms, Spermatic cords, Kidneys, Urine).

GERD (Gastro-esophageal-reflux disease)
   - Natrum mur. 6x
   - Calc.sulph. 6x
   - Calc.flor. 6x

GESTATIONAL DIABETES (See Diabetes)

GINGIVITIS (inflammation of gums) (See Gums)

GLANDS - DISEASES OF LYMPH NODES
Inflammation (Lymhadenitis)
    Natrum sulph. 6x
    Kali.sulph. 6x
    Calc.sulph. 6x
Soft, enlarged lymph glands
    Kali.phos. 6x
    Kali.sulph. 6x
    Calc.sulph. 6x
Stony hard, enlarged lymph glands
    Natrum sulph. 6x
    Kali.sulph. 6x
    Calc.sulph. 6x

GLAUCOMA (See Eye diseases)

GLEET (See Gonorrhoea)

GLOMERULAR FILTRATION RATE (GFR), decreased
    Kali.sulph. 6x
    Calc.sulph. 6x
    Silicea 6x

GLOSSITIS (Inflammation of tongue) (See Tongue)

GOITRE
1. Endemic goiter (due to iodine deficiency)
    Natrum sulph. 6x
    Kali.sulph. 6x
    Calc.sulph. 6x
2. Hyperthyroidism, exophthalmic goitre
    Natrum mur. 6x
    Kali.mur. 6x
    Calc.sulph. 6x

3. Hypothyroidism (Myxoedema)
        Ferrum phos 6x
        Natrum mur. 6x
        Calc.sulph. 6x
(See Myxoedema also)

GONORRHOEA *(Sexually transmitted disease of genito-urinary system, caused by gonococcus bacteria).*

1. Acute inflammation
        Kali.sulph. 6x
        Calc.sulph. 6x
        Silicea 6x
2. Adenitis, lymhangitis in genital region
        Kali.mur. 6x
        Kali.sulph. 6x
        Calc.sulph. 6x
3. Chronic gonorrhoea
        Natrum sulph. 6x
        Kali.sulph. 6x
        Calc.sulph. 6x

GONORRHOEA - Other organs involved

1. Arthritis, rheumatism-gonorrheal
        Kali.sulph. 6x
        Calc.sulph. 6x
        Silicea 6x
2. Ophthalmia, neonatorum (in newborn)
        Natrum sulph. 6x
        Kali.sulph. 6x
        Calc.sulph. 6x

3. Orchitis, epididymitis - gonorrheal

  Natrum sulph. 6x
  Kali sulph. 6x
  Calc.sulph. 6x

4. Prostatic involvement - gonorrheal

  Kali.sulph. 6x
  Calc.sulph. 6x
  Silicea 6x

5. Stricture, Urethra - gonorrhoeal

  Natrum sulph. 6x
  Kali.sulph. 6x
  Calc.sulph. 6x

6. Suppression of gonorrhea - ill-effects

  Natrum sulph. 6x
  Calc.sulph. 6x
  Kali.sulph. 6x

GONORRHOEA - DISCHARGE

1. Bloody dscharge

  Calc.sulph. 6x
  Kali.sulph. 6x
  Silicea 6x

2. Milky, glairy, mucus discharge

  Natrum sulph. 6x
  Kali.sulph. 6x
  Calc.sulph. 6x

3. Muco-purulent, yellowish-green pus

  Natrum sulph. 6x
  Kali.sulph. 6x
  Calc.sulph. 6x

GOUT (Hyperuricemia or increased uric acid in blood)

1. Acute gout

  Natrum sulph. 6x
  Kali.sulph. 6x
  Calc.flor. 6x

2. Chronic gout
        Kali.sulph. 6x
        Calc.sulph. 6x
        Silicea 6x

GRAVE'S DISEASE (Hyperthyroidism) (See Goitre)

GROWTH HORMONE - DEFICIENCY
        Kali.phos. 6x
        Natrum sulph. 6x
        Calc.sulph. 6x

GROWTH, STUNTED (See Height also)
        Calc.phos. 6x
        Kali.sulph. 6x
        Calc.flor. 6x

GUMS
1. Bleeding, easily
        Ferrum phos 6x
        Calc.sulph. 6x
        Silicea 6x
2. Bleeding, excessive, after tooth extraction
        Calc.phos. 6x
        Ferrum phos 6x
        Calc.flor. 6x
3. Inflammation (gumboil)
        Kali.sulph. 6x
        Calc.sulph. 6x
        Silicea 6x
4. Pain, after tooth extraction
        Kali.phos. 6x
        Kali.mur. 6x
        Calc.sulph. 6x
5. Pain, sore, sensitive, gingivitis
        Kali.sulph. 6x
        Calc.sulph. 6x
        Silicea 6x

6. Pyorrhoea alveolaris (pus in bony socket of tooth)
   - Kali.sulph. 6x
   - Calc.sulph. 6x
   - Silicea 6x

7. Scorbutic (soft, spongy, receding gums)
   - Natrum mur. 6x
   - Kali.sulph. 6x
   - Calc.sulph. 6x

8. Ulceration of gums
   - Natrum mur. 6x
   - Kali.mur. 6x
   - Calc.sulph. 6x

H

HAIR FALLING
1. General formula
   - Natrum mur. 6x
   - Kali.mur. 6x
   - Calc.sulph. 6x
2. After some acute disease
   - Kali.phos. 6x
   - Natrum sulph. 6x
   - Calc.sulph. 6x
3. Bunches of hair fall with combing or brushing
   - Ferrum phos 6x
   - Natrum sulph. 6x
   - Calc.sulph. 6x
4. Climacteric (menopause), during
   - Kali.phos. 6x
   - Kali.mur. 6x
   - Calc.sulph. 6x
5. Falling in spots or in patches
   - Natrum sulph. 6x
   - Kali.phos. 6x
   - Calc.sulph. 6x
6. Familial hair falling
   - Kali.mur. 6x
   - Kali.sulph. 6x
   - Calc.sulph. 6x
7. Grief - hair falling, due to
   - Kali.sulph. 6x
   - Calc.sulph. 6x
   - Silicea 6x
8. Headache - due to
   - Natrum mur. 6x
   - Natrum sulph. 6x
   - Kali.mur. 6x

9. Lactation - during
 - Natrum mur. 6x
 - Natrum sulph. 6x
 - Kali.mur. 6x

10. Mental work, studies - after
 - Kali.phos. 6x
 - Kali.mur. 6x
 - Calc.sulph. 6x

HAIR

1. Absent or deficient growth, on face of males
 - Kali.phos. 6x
 - Natrum mur. 6x
 - Calc.sulph. 6x

2. Dry and lusterless hair
 - Kali.phos. 6x
 - Natrum sulph. 6x
 - Calc.sulph. 6x

3. Split into two parts, at the end of hair (split hair)
 - Kali.mur. 6x
 - Calc.sulph. 6x
 - Natrum mur. 6x

4. Tangled hair, difficult to brush or separate
 - Natrum mur. 6x
 - Kali.mur. 6x
 - Calc.sulph. 6x

5. Thin, silky hair, break easily
 - Natrum mur. 6x
 - Kali.sulph. 6x
 - Calc.sulph. 6x

6. Unwanted hair, on face of females (Hirsutism)
 - Calc.phos. 6x
 - Calc.sulph. 6x
 - Natrum sulph. 6x

HAIR TWIRLING - plucking the hair (trichotillomania)

Natrum mur.	6x
Kali.mur.	6x
Calc.sulph.	6x

HANDS
1. Arthritis (See Arthritis)
2. Carpel tunnel syndrome (See Carpel tunnel syndrome)
3. Dupuytren's contracture

Kali.phos.	6x
Natrum sulph.	6x
Calc.flor.	6x

4. Ganglion, cyst (See Ganglion)
5. Hot hands, palms

Calc.phos.	6x
Ferrum phos.	6x
Natrum mur.	6x

6. Muscle wasting or atrophy

Natrum sulph.	6x
Calc.sulph.	6x
Silicea	6x

7. Numbness (See Numbness)
8. Pain and stiffness in hands

Natrum sulph.	6x
Kali.sulph.	6x
Calc.sulph.	6x

9. Paralysis of hand

Kali.phos.	6x
Kali.sulph.	6x
Calc.sulph.	6x

10. Raynaurd's disease (See Raynaud's disease)
11. Rheumatoid arthritis (See Rheumatoid arthritis)
12. Hands-palms, sweating

Kali.phos.	6x
Natrum sulph.	6x
Calc.sulph.	6x

13. Swelling of hands
    - Natrum sulph. 6x
    - Kali.sulph. 6x
    - Calc.sulph. 6x
14. Tendinitis (See Tendinitis)
15. Teno-synovitis (See Teno-synovitis)
16. Tremors (See Parkinson's disease)
17. Trigger finger (Finger is stuck in bent position due to hardening of the tendons of finger in synovial sheath)
    - Kali.mur. 6x
    - Kali.sulph. 6x
    - Calc.flor. 6x

HAND-FOOT-AND-MOUTH DISEASE (A disease in young children caused by coxsackie virus which produces soreness of mouth and rash on hands and feet)
- Natrum mur. 6x
- Calc.sulph. 6x
- Silicea 6x

HANGOVER
- Natrum sulph. 6x
- Calc.sulph. 6x
- Silicea 6x

HAY FEVER (sneezing, running nose and congestion of respiratoty system caused by allergic response to airborne substances like pollen, in Spring and harvesting season)
- Kali.phos. 6x
- Natrum mur. 6x
- Kali.sulph. 6x
- Calc.sulph. 6x

HEADACHE – CAUSES
1. General formula
   - Kali.phos. 6x
   - Mag.phos. 6x
   - Natrum mur. 6x

2. Catarrh, due to
- Kali.phos. 6x
- Natrum sulph. 6x
- Kali sulph. 6x

3. Catarrh - suppressed
- Kali.phos. 6x
- Kali.sulph. 6x
- Calc.sulph. 6x

4. Constipation
- Kali.phos. 6x
- Natrum sulph. 6x
- Calc.sulph. 6x

5. Emotional disturbances
- Kali.phos. 6x
- Natrum mur. 6x
- Calc.sulph. 6x

6. Eye-strain
- Calc.phos. 6x
- Kali.phos. 6x
- Natrum mur. 6x

7. Castro-intestinal derangements
- Kali.phos. 6x
- Natrum mur. 6x
- Kali.mur. 6x

8. Mental exertion or exhaustion
- Kali.phos. 6x
- Kali.mur. 6x
- Calc.sulph. 6x

9. Sinusitis, due to
- Natrum sulph. 6x
- Kali.sulph. 6x
- Calc.sulph. 6x

10. Sunlight or heat
- Mag.phos. 6x
- Natrum sulph. 6x
- Calc.sulph. 6x

11. Tobacco

Kali.phos.	6x
Natrum sulph.	6x
Calc.sulph.	6x

HEADACHE – LOCATION
1. Frontal, forehead region

Kali.sulph.	6x
Calc.sulph.	6x
Silicea	6x

2. Occipitial pain (back of head)

Kali.phos.	6x
Natrum sulph.	6x
Calc.sulph.	6x

3. Temples pain

Natrum mur.	6x
Kali.sulph.	6x
Calc.sulph.	6x

4. Vertex pain (Crown of head)

Mag.phos.	6x
Kali.mur.	6x
Calc.sulph.	6x

HEADACHE – TYPES
1. Anaemic headache

Ferrum phos	6x
Natrum mur.	6x
Calc.sulph.	6x

2. Chronic headache

Natrum mur.	6x
Calc.sulph.	6x
Silicea	6x

3. Chronic headache of, sedentary persons

Calc.sulph.	6x
Kali.phos.	6x
Natrum sulph.	6x

4. Cluster headache

    Kali.phos.   6x
    Natrum mur.   6x
    Calc.sulph.   6x

5. Gastric, bilious headache

    Natrum sulph.   6x
    Kali.sulph.   6x
    Calc.flor.   6x

6. Hysterical headache

    Kali.phos.   6x
    Natrum sulph.   6x
    Calc.sulph.   6x

7. School girls, headache

    Natrum sulph.   6x
    Kali.sulph.   6x
    Calc.sulph.   6x

8. Students, headache

    Kali.phos.   6x
    Kali.sulph.   6x
    Calc.sulph.   6x

9. Tension headache

    Kali.phos.   6x
    Natrum sulph.   6x
    Calc.sulph.   6x

HEADACHE – CONCOMITANTS

1. Arteries, pulsating with headache

    Natrum mur.   6x
    Kali.mur.   6x
    Calc.sulph.   6x

2. Constipation with headache
   - Natrum sulph. 6x
   - Kali.sulph. 6x
   - Silicea 6x
3. Exhaustion, weakness with headache
   - Kali.phos. 6x
   - Calc.sulph. 6x
   - Silicea 6x
4. Irritability with headache
   - Kali.phos. 6x
   - Natrum mur. 6x
   - Calc.sulph. 6x
5. Visual disturbances, before or during headache
   - Kali.phos. 6x
   - Natrum sulph. 6x
   - Calc.sulph. 6x

HEAD INJURy AND AFTER-EFFECTS
- Natrum sulph. 6x
- Kali.sulph. 6x
- Calc.sulph. 6x

HEART BURN (See Dyspepsia)

HEART DISEASES
1. Action of heart - violent, laoured
   - Kali.phos. 6x
   - Natrum mur. 6x
   - Silicea 6x
2. Cardiac arrhythmia, with missing beats and fainting
   - Kali.phos. 6x
   - Natrum sulph. 6x
   - Calc.sulph. 6x
3. Cornary artey disease (See Coronary)
   - Calc.phos. 6x
   - Kali.phos. 6x
   - Kali.mur. 3x

4. Debility, weakness of heart
   - Kali.phos. 6x
   - Ferrum phos 6x
   - Natrum sulph. 6x
5. Enlarged (hypertrophied heart)
   - Kali.phos. 6x
   - Natrum sulph. 6x
   - Calc.sulph. 6x
6. Fatty degeneration of heart
   - Kali.sulph. 6x
   - Calc.sulph. 6x
   - Silicea 6x
7. Heart failure
   - Kali.phos. 6x
   - Natrum sulph. 6x
   - Calc.sulph. 6x
8. Nervous, emotional causes
   - Kali.phos. 6x
   - Natrum sulph. 6x
   - Calc.sulph. 6x
9. With dropsy of legs or feet
   - Kali.mur. 6x
   - Kali.sulph. 6x
   - Calc.sulph. 6x
10. Inflammation of heart (Endocarditis)
    - Kali.phos. 6x
    - Natrum sulph. 6x
    - Kali sulph. 6x
11. Myocardial infaction (heart attack)
    - Kali.phos. 3x
    - Natrum sulph. 6x
    - Calc.sulph. 6x

Dose: Reapeat after every 15 minutes, till pain subsides. After that use it 4-6 times a day.

Pericarditis
1. Acute pericarditis
    - Kali.mur. 6x
    - Kali.sulph. 6x
    - Calc.sulph. 6x
2. Chronic pericarditis
    - Kali.sulph. 6x
    - Calc.sulph. 6x
    - Silicea 6x

Pain - Heart
1. Angina pectoris
    - Calc.sulph. 6x
    - Calc.flor. 6x
    - Silicea 6x
2. From organic heart disease
    - Kali.mur. 6x
    - Kali.sulph. 6x
    - Calc.sulph. 6x
3. From tobacco smoking
    - Kali.phos. 6x
    - Kali.mur. 6x
    - Silicea 6x
4. Praecordial oppression, anxiety, heaviness
    - Calc.sulph. 6x
    - Calc.flor. 6x
    - Silicea 6x
5. Shooting down left shoulder, arm to fingers
    - Kali.sulph. 6x
    - Calc.sulph. 6x
    - Silicea 6x

Palpitations - Heart
1. General formula
    - Calc.sulph. 6x
    - Calc.flor. 6x
    - Silicea 6x

2. Anaemia, or due to vital drains
   - Natrum mur. 6x
   - Kali.sulph. 6x
   - Calc.sulph. 6x
3. Dyspepsia, with
   - Calc.sulph. 6x
   - Calc.flor. 6x
   - Silicea 6x
4. Tobacco
   - Kali.phos. 6x
   - Kali.mur. 6x
   - Silicea 6x

Palpitations - Concomitants
1. Dyspnoea (breathlessness)
   - Calc.sulph. 6x
   - Kali.sulph. 6x
   - Silicea 6x
2. With flatulence (gas)
   - Kali.sulph. 6x
   - Calc.sulph. 6x
   - Silicea
3. With pain, praecordial (region of heart)
   - Calc.sulph. 6x
   - Kali.sulph. 6x
   - Silicea 6x
4. With sleeplessness
   - Silicea 6x
   - Calc.sulph. 6x
   - Kali sulph. 6x

Palpitations - Aggravation
1. After eating
   - Kali.phos. 6x
   - Natrum sulph. 6x
   - Calc.sulph. 6x

2. From lying on left side
  Kali.phos. 6x
  Kali.sulph. 6x
  Calc.sulph. 6x
3. From lying on right side
  Natrum mur. 6x
  Kali.mur. 6x
  Calc.flor. 6x
4. Rheumatic heart disease
  Kali.sulph. 6x
  Calc.sulph. 6x
  Silicea 6x
5. Valvular diseases – HEART (See Valvular diseases)

HEAT RASH
  Natrum sulph. 6x
  Calc.sulph. 6x
  Silicea 6x

HEEL - PAIN
1. Arhtritis - heel
  Ferrum phos 6x
  Kali.sulph. 6x
  Calc.sulph. 6x
2. Bursitis - heel
  Kali.phos. 6x
  Natrum sulph. 6x
  Calc.sulph. 6x
3. Calcaneal spur (sharp outgrowth under heel bone)
  Kali.sulph. 6x
  Calc.sulph. 6x
  Calc.flor. 6x
  Silicea 6x
4. Stress fracture or injury - heel bone
  Kali.phos. 6x
  Natrum mur. 6x
  Calc.sulph. 6x

HEIGHT-STUNTED
                        Kali.phos.   6x
                        Calc.sulph.   6x
                        Natrum sulph. 6x

HEMANGIOMA
1. General formula
                        Kali.phos.   6x
                        Natrum sulph. 6x
                        Calc.sulph.   6x
2. External hemangioma (on skin), in newborn
                        Calc.sulph.   6x
                        Calc.flor.   6x
                        Silicea   6x
3. Hemangioma, Internal hemangioma - Brain
                        Silicea   6x
                        Kali.sulph.   6x
                        Calc.sulph.   6x

4. Hemangioma - Liver, mostly drug induced
                        Calc.sulph.   6x
                        Silicea   6x
                        Kali.sulph.   6x

HEMATEMESIS (Vomiting of blood from stomach)
                        Kali.sulph.   6x
                        Calc.sulph.   6x
                        Silicea   6x

HEMATURIA (blood in urine)
1. General formula
                        Natrum sulph. 6x
                        Kali.sulph.   6x
                        Calc.sulph.   6x
2. Gross hematuria
                        Kali.mur.   6x
                        Kali.sulph.   6x
                        Calc.sulph.   6x

3. Microscopic hemturia

Calc.phos.	6x
Kali.mur.	6x
Calc.sulph.	6x

Note: Also find and treat the causes like urinary tract infection, kidney stone, kidney diseases and others.

HEMOGLOBINURIA

Natrum mur.	6x
Kali.mur.	6x
Calc.sulph.	6x

HEMOPHILIA

Calc.phos.	6x
Kali.phos.	6x
Natrum sulph.	6x

HEMOPTYSIS (Bleeding from lungs with cough)

1. Bright red blood

Calc.phos.	6x
Ferrum phos	6x
Calc.sulph.	6x

2. Due to tuberculosis

Kali.sulph.	6x
Calc.sulph.	6x
Silicea	6x

3. Mitral stenosis cases

Kali.sulph.	6x
Calc.sulph.	6x
Calc.flor.	6x

4. Due to other causes

Kali.phos.	6x
Kali.sulph.	6x
Calc.sulph.	6x

HEMORRHAGES (Bleeding from any part of body)

1. General formula

Kali.sulph.	6x
Calc.sulph.	6x
Silicea	6x

2. From trauma
   - Calc.phos. 6x
   - Ferrum phos 6x
   - Natrum sulph. 6x
3. Blood, bright red
   - Kali.sulph. 6x
   - Calc.sulph. 6x
   - Silicea 6x
4. Blood, clotted, partly fluid
   - Kali.phos. 6x
   - Natrum sulph. 6x
   - Calc.sulph. 6x
5. Blood, dark, clotted
   - Kali sulph. 6x
   - Calc.sulph. 6x
   - Calc.flor. 6x
6. Tubercular
   - Calc.phos. 6x
   - Kali.sulph. 6x
   - Calc.sulph. 6x
7. With valvular disease of heart
   - Natrum sulph. 6x
   - Kali.sulph. 6x
   - Calc.sulph. 6x

Vicarious bleeding (cyclical bleeding from orgns other than the uterus during menstrual cycle). Examples: From nose, mouth, eyes (red tears).
   - Kali.mur. 6x
   - Kali.sulph. 6x
   - Calc.sulph. 6x

HEMORRHOIDS, PILES
1. General formula

Calc.phos.	6x
Ferrum phos	6x
Natrum sulph.	6x
Calc.sulph.	6x
Calc.flor.	6x

2. Bleeding piles

Natrum sulph.	6x
Kali.sulph.	6x
Calc.sulph.	6x
Silicea	

3. Non-bleeding piles or internal piles

Natrum sulph.	6x
Kali.sulph.	6x
Calc.sulph.	6x

4. In resistant cases

Kali.sulph.	6x
Calc.sulph.	6x
Calc.flor.	6x
Silicea	6x

HEPATITIS (See Liver, inflammation)

HERNIA
1. Epigastric hernia

Natrum sulph.	6x
Kali.mur.	6x
Kali sulph.	6x

2. Femoral hernia

Kali.phos.	6x
Mag.phos.	6x
Nat.phos.	6x

3. Hiatus hernia

	Natrum sulph.	6x
	Kali.mur.	6x
	Calc.sulph.	6x

4. Incisional hernia (due to surgical operation)

	Calc.phos.	6x
	Kali.sulph.	6x
	Calc.sulph.	6x

5. Inguinal hernia

	Natrum sulph.	6x
	Kali.sulph.	6x
	Calc.sulph.	6x

6. Scrotal hernia

	Calc.sulph.	6x
	Kali.mur.	6x
	Calc.flor.	6x

7. Umbilical hernia

	Calc.sulph.	6x
	Calc.flor.	6x
	Silicea	6x

HERPES SIMPLEX

	Natrum sulph.	6x
	Kali.sulph.	6x
	Calc.sulph.	6x

HERPES ZOSTER (Shingles)

	Natrum sulph.	6x
	Kali.mur.	6x
	Kali sulph.	6x

HICCUPS

	Kali.phos.	6x
	Kali.mur.	6x
	Calc.sulph.	6x

HIGH BLOOD PRESSURE (See Hypertension)

HIP JOINT - ARTHRITIS
            Natrum sulph.   6x
            Kali.sulph.   6x
            Calc.sulph.   6x
            Silicea   6x

HIRSCHPRUNG DISEASE (Absence of nerve cells in colon by bith)
            Kali.phos.   6x
            Natrum sulph.   6x
            Calc.sulph.   6x

HIRSUTISM (Unwatnted hair on face of females)
            Calc.phos.   6x
            Calc.sulph.   6x
            Natrum sulph.   6x

HISTOPLASMOSIS (Fungal disease caused by histoplasma)
            Kali.phos.   6x
            Natrum sulph.   6x
            Calc.sulph.   6x

HIVES (Nettlerash, Urticaria) (See urticaria also)
            Natrum mur.   6x
            Kali.sulph.   6x
            Calc.sulph.   6x

HORMONE IMBALANCE (Females)
            Kali.phos.   6x
            Natrum sulph.   6x
            Calc.sulph.   6x

HORMONE IMBALANCE (Males)
            Natrum mur.   6x
            Kali.mur.   6x
            Silicea   6x

HORNER'S SYNDROME

    a. Kali.phos. 6x
       Natrum sulph. 6x
       Calc.sulph. 6x

    b. Kali.sulph. 6x
       Calc.sulph. 6x
       Silicea 6x

(See Laryngitis also)

HODGKIN'S DISEASE (Pseudo-leukemia)

    Kali.phos. 6x
    Natrum sulph. 6x
    Kali.mur. 6x

HOUSEMAID'S KNEE (Pre-patellar bursitis)

    Natrum sulph. 6x
    Kali.sulph. 6x
    Calc.sulph. 6x

HUMAN IMMUNODEFICIENCY VIRUS (HIV)

    Kali.phos. 6x
    Natrum sulph. 6x
    Kali.sulph. 6x
    Calc.sulph. 6x

HUNTINGTON'S DISEASE

    Kali.phos. 6x
    Natrum mur. 6x
    Calc.sulph. 6x

H. PYLORI INFECTION

    Kali.phos. 6x
    Natrum mur. 6x
    Natrum sulph. 6x
    Calc.sulph. 6x

HYDROCELE

    Kali.phos. 6x
    Kali.sulph. 6x

Calc.sulph. 6x

HYDROCEPHALUS (Abnormal and excess collection of fluid in the ventricles of brain)

Natrum sulph. 6x
Kali.sulph. 6x
Calc.sulph. 6x

HYPEREMESIS GRAVIDARUM (Severe nausea and vomiting during pregnancy)

Kali.phos. 12x
Natrum sulph. 6x
Calc.sulph. 6x

HYPERGLYCEMIA (See Diabetes)

HYPERMETROPIA (Far-sightedness or weak near vision)

Kali.phos. 6x
Natrum mur. 6x
Calc.sulph. 6x

MYOPIA (Near-sightedness, weak distant vision)

Ferrum phos 6x
Natrum mur. 6x
Kali.mur. 6x

HYPER-PARATHYROIDISM

Kali.phos. 6x
Nat.phos. 6x
Natrum sulph. 6x

HYPER-PROLACTINEMIA

Natrum sulph. 6x
Kali.sulph. 6x
Calc.flor. 6x

HYPERTENSION
1. Primary hypertension

Kali.phos. 6x
Natrum mur. 6x
Kali.mur. 6x

2. Secondary hypertension (due to drugs or other causes).
a. Drugs (estrogen, steroids, etc.)

Natrum mur. 6x
Kali.mur. 6x

b. Endocrine or hormonal disorders

  Calc.sulph. 6x
  Natrum sulph. 6x
  Kali.sulph. 6x
  Calc.sulph. 6x

c. Pregnancy (Pre-eclampsia, toxemia)

  Calc.phos. 6x
  Ferrum phos 6x
  Kali.phos. 6x

d. Renal infection

  Kali.sulph. 6x
  Calc.sulph. 6x
  Calc.flor. 6x

d. Renal artery stenosis

  Natrum mur. 6x
  Natrum sulph. 6x
  Kali.mur. 6x

HYPERTENSION – Concomitant diseases

1. With anxiety, headache, numbness and sleeplessness

  Natrum mur. 6x
  Kali.mur. 6x
  Calc.sulph. 6x

2. With palpitation, angina pectoris, sleep problems

  Natrum mur. 6x
  Kali.mur. 6x
  Calc.sulph. 6x

3. With anxiety, neuroses, headaches, muscular pain and extreme depression

  Kali.sulph. 6x
  Calc.sulph. 6x
  Calc.flor. 6x

HYPERTHERMIA (Extreme heat of body)

  Natrum sulph. 6x
  Kali.phos. 6x
  Calc.sulph. 6x

HYPERVENTILATION

Calc.sulph.	6x
Kali.phos.	6x
Natrum sulph.	6x

HYPOCHONDRIASIS

Natrum sulph.	6x
Calc.sulph.	6x
Kali.phos.	6x

HYPOTHERMIA (Extreme coldness of body)

Calc.phos.	6x
Kali.phos.	6x
Natrum sulph.	6x

HYPERTHYROIDISM

Natrum mur.	6x
Kali.mur.	6x
Calc.sulph.	6x

HYPOTENSION

Kali.phos.	6x
Natrum mur.	6x
Natrum sulph.	6x
Silicea	6x

HYPOTHYROIDISM

Ferrum phos	6x
Natrum mur.	6x
Calc.sulph.	6x

HYSTERIA

Kali.phos.	6x
Natrum sulph.	6x
Calc.sulph.	6x

I

IBD (Crohn's disease and ulcerative colitis).
(See Irritable bowel disease)
IBS (See Irritable bowel syndrome)
ICHTHYOSIS (Fish scales diseases, Xeroderma)

Natrum sulph.	6x
Kali.sulph.	6x
Calc.sulph.	6x

IMMUNE SYSTEM BOOSTER

Kali.phos.	6x
Natrum sulph.	6x
Calc.sulph.	6x

IMPETIGO

Ferrum phos	6x
Natrum sulph.	6x
Calc.sulph.	6x
Silicea	6x

IMPOTENCE (See Penis, Emissions, Sexual disorders, Spermatorrhoea, Semen, Weakness)

1. Erectile dysfunction (ED)

Kali.phos.	6x
Natrum mur.	6x
Kali.sulph.	6x
Calc.sulph.	6x

2. Premature ejaculation

Natrum sulph.	6x
Kali.sulph.	6x
Calc.sulph.	6x

3. Weak erections

Kali.phos.	6x
Natrum sulph.	6x
Kali.sulph.	6x
Calc.sulph.	6x

INDIGESTION (See Dyspepsia)
INFANTS

1. Abdominal colic
   - Kali.sulph. 6x
   - Calc.sulph. 6x
   - Silicea 6x

2. Abdominal distention
   - Silicea 6x
   - Calc.sulph. 6x
   - Kali.sulph. 6x

3. Anemia
   - Calc.phos. 6x
   - Natrum mur. 6x
   - Silicea 6x

4. Appetite, poor
   - a. Nat.phos. 6x
     - Natrum sulph. 6x
     - Calc.sulph. 6x
   - b. Calc.phos. 6x
     - Natrum mur. 6x
     - Natrum mur. 6x

5. Birth apnoea with bluish skin
   - Kali.phos. 6x
   - Natrum sulph. 6x
   - Calc.sulph. 6x

6. Birth injuries
   - Calc.sulph. 6x
   - Calc.flor. 6x
   - Silicea 6x

7. Bronchitis
   - (See Bronchitis)

8. Burping, difficult
   - Kali.phos. 6x
   - Calc.sulph. 6x
   - Silicea 6x

9. Common cold and flu (See Cold and Flu)

10. Constipation

Kali.phos.	6x
Kali.sulph.	6x
Calc.sulph.	6x

11. Constipation

Natrum sulph.	6x
Natrum mur.	6x
Silicea	6x

    Dose: Give once or twice daily.

12. Cough

Natrum sulph.	6x
Kali.sulph.	6x
Calc.sulph.	6x

13. Cyanosis (See Cyanosis)

14. Delayed milestones of development

Ferrum phos	6x
Natrum mur.	6x
Calc.sulph.	6x

15. Diaper rash

Kali.phos.	6x
Natrum sulph.	6x
Calc.sulph.	6x

16. Diarrhea (See Diarrhea)
17. Dysentery (See Dysentery)
18. Ear infection (See Ear)
19. Fever (See Fever)
20. Gas in abdomen, discomfort

Natrum sulph.	6x
Calc.sulph.	6x
Kali sulph.	6x

21. Jaundice (See Jundice)
22. Laryngomalacia

Kali.phos.	6x
Natrum sulph.	6x
Calc.sulph.	6x

23. Low birth weight

    Natrum mur. 6x
    Kali.sulph. 6x
    Calc.sulph. 6x

24. Marasmus, Kwashiorkor

    Calc.phos. 6x
    Kali.phos. 6x
    Natrum mur. 6x

25. Nasal obstruction, congestion, mouth breathing

    Calc.sulph. 6x
    Calc.flor. 6x
    Silicea 6x

26. Pneumonia

    Natrum sulph. 6x
    Calc.sulph. 6x
    Silicea 6x

27. Restlessness

    Calc.phos. 6x
    Kali.phos. 6x
    Natrum sulph. 6x

28. Respiratory distress

    Ferrum phos 6x
    Natrum sulph. 6x
    Calc.sulph. 6x

29. Sleep problems

    Natrum sulph. 6x
    Kali.sulph. 6x
    Calc.sulph. 6x

30. Teething problems   (See Dentiotion)

31. Throat infection   (See Pharyngitis)
32. Thrush in mouth

    Kali.mur. 6x
    Kali.sulph. 6x
    Calc.sulph. 6x

33. Vomiting or throwing up milk

Natrum sulph.	6x
Calc.sulph.	6x
Silicea	6x

34. Weeping or crying

Kali.phos.	6x
Natrum sulph.	6x
Calc.sulph.	6x

Note: Treat rest of the diseases, as in respective sections.

INFERTILITY (See Sterility – Male, Female)

INFLAMMATION (Any part or organ of body)

Kali.mur.	6x
Kali.sulph.	6x
Calc.sulph.	6x

INFLAMATORY BOWEL SYNDROME (IBS)

Kali.phos.	6x
Natrum sulph.	6x
Calc.sulph.	6x

INFLUENZA - all types (see flu, influenza, coryza, cough, fever, pharyngitis, bronchitis, viral diseases, severe acute respiratory syndrome, asphyxia, cyanosis, avian influenza, septicemia, bird flu, cyanosis, multiple organ dysfunction syndrome, bronchospam, cough, pneumonia, swine flu, coma, blood clotting, clotting of blood and oxygen low saturation and other relevant symptoms).

1. General formula for prevention - all types of influenza

Kali.phos.	6x
Natrum sulph.	6x
Kali.sulph.	6x
Calc.sulph.	6x

Dose: one tablet daily for one month. One tablet on alternate days, below 12 years age, for one month.

2. General formula for treatment

Kali.phos.	6x
Kali.sulph.	6x
Calc.sulph.	6x

3. Breathing difficulty with influenza
    Kali.phos. 6x
    Kali.sulph. 6x
    Calc.sulph. 6x
4. Blood clotting tendency, with
    Natrum sulph. 6x
    Kali.sulph. 6x
    Calc.sulph. 6x
(See blood clotting and hemorrahge also)
5. Debility with or after influenza
    Kali.sulph. 6x
    Calc.sulph. 6x
    Silicea 6x
6. H1N1 influenza (Bird flu)
    Kali.sulph. 6x
    Calc.sulph. 6x
    Calc.flor. 6x
    Silicea 6x
7. Seasonal flu (prevention and treatment)
    Kali.phos. 6x
    Kali.sulph. 6x
    Calc.sulph. 6x
Prevention: Once daily for one month.
Treatment: 3 to 4 times daily.

8. Swine flu in human (H3 N2 virus)
    Kali.sulph. 6x
    Calc.sulph. 6x
    Calc.flor. 6x
    Silicea 6x

INGROWN TOE-NAIL (See Nails)
INJURIES and after-effects
1. General formula - injuries and after-effects
    Kali.sulph. 6x
    Calc.sulph. 6x
    Calc.flor. 6x

2. Bone injuries
 - Calc.phos. 6x
 - Calc.sulph. 6x
 - Calc.flor. 6x
3. Chronic effects of injuries
 - Kali.phos. 6x
 - Natrum sulph. 6x
 - Calc.sulph. 6x
4. Mental symptoms, from injuries
 - Kali.phos. 6x
 - Natrum mur. 6x
 - Calc.sulph. 6x
5. Parts, rich in sentient nerves such as fingers, toes
 - Kali.phos. 6x
 - Natrum sulph. 6x
 - Calc.sulph. 6x
6. Surgical operation and its after-effects
 - Kali.phos. 6x
 - Natrum sulph. 6x
 - Calc.sulph. 6x

INSANITY (See Depression, Mania, Memory, Delirium, Moods, eg. anxiety, apathetic, aversion).
 - Kali.phos. 6x
 - Natrum sulph. 6x
 - Calc.sulph. 6x

INSECT BITES (Wasp, bee, mosquito, spider, scorpion)
 - Kali.phos. 6x
 - Kali.sulph. 6x
 - Calc.sulph. 6x

Dose: Give after every five minutes, till the pain stops. After that give 3 or 4 times daily.
Exernal application: Natrum mur. 3x or 6x mixed in water.

INSOMNIA   (See Sleeplessness)

INTERMITTENT FEVER

Natrum mur. 6x
Kali.mur. 6x
Calc.sulph. 6x

INTERTRIGO (Chaffing in the folds of skin)

Natrum mur. 6x
Kali.sulph. 6x
Calc.sulph. 6x

INTESTINES
1. Intussusception, obstruction of intestine

Kali.phos. 6x
Kali.mur. 6x
Calc.sulph. 6x

Dose: Give after every 10 minutes; after 10 doses, increase the interval.

2. Ulceration-intestines

Natrum sulph. 6x
Kali.sulph. 6x
Calc.sulph. 6x

IRIS
1. Iritis (inflammation of iris)

Ferrum phos 6x
Calc.sulph. 6x
Silicea 6x

2. Iritis, rheumatic

Natrum sulph. 6x
Kali.sulph. 6x
Calc.sulph. 6x

3. Iritis, traumatic

Kali.phos. 6x
Natrum sulph. 6x
Kali sulph. 6x

4. Proplapse of iris

      Kali.phos. 6x
      Kali.sulph. 6x
      Calc.sulph. 6x

IRON DEFICIENCY ANEMIA

      Ferrum phos 6x
      Natrum mur. 6x
      Silicea 6x

IRRITABLE BOWEL DISEASE (Crohn's disease and ulcerative colitis)

  a. Calc.sulph. 6x
    Natrum sulph. 6x
    Natrum mur. 6x

  b. Calc. phos. 6x
    Natsrum sulph. 6x
    Ferrum phos 6x

IRRITABLE BOWEL SYNDROME (IBS)

      Kali.phos. 6x
      Natrum sulph. 6x
      Kali.sulph. 6x
      Calc.sulph. 6x

ITCHING (See pruritis, eczema)

J

JAUNDICE (icterus) (See Liver, Hepatitis also)
1. Acute jaundice
   - Ferrum phos   6x
   - Natrum sulph. 6x
   - Calc.sulph.   6x
2. Chronic jaundice
   - Natrum sulph. 6x
   - Kali.sulph.   6x
   - Calc.sulph.   6x
3. Hemolytic jaundice
   - Natrum mur.   6x
   - Kali.sulph.   6x
   - Calc.sulph.   6x
4. Infant is born with jaundice (pathological jaundice)
   - Natrum sulph. 6x
   - Kali.sulph.   6x
   - Calc.sulph.   6x
5. Jaundice appears few days after birth (physiological jaundice)
   - Natrum sulph. 6x
   - Calc.sulph.   6x
   - Silicea   6x

JAWS
1. Caries, necrosis
   - Kali.phos.   6x
   - Natrum sulph. 6x
   - Calc.sulph.   6x
2. Cracking sound - temporo-mandiular joint
   - Calc.phos.   6x
   - Kali.phos.   6x
   - Calc.sulph.   6x
3. Dislocated easily-TM joint
   - Kali.phos.   6x
   - Natrum sulph. 6x
   - Calc.sulph.   6x

4. Growth, swelling in jaw

	Natrum mur.	6x
	Kali.mur.	6x
	Calc.flor.	6x

5. Pain in jaws

	Kali.phos.	6x
	Natrum sulph.	6x
	Kali sulph.	6x

6. Pain in TM joint

	Kali.phos.	6x
	Kali.sulph.	6x
	Calc.sulph.	6x

7. Stiffness (Trismus, lockjaw)

	Kali.phos.	6x
	Natrum sulph.	6x
	Calc.sulph.	6x

JAW, UPPER
Maxillary sinus, diseases of

	Kali.mur.	6x
	Calc.sulph.	6x
	Silicea	6x

JET - LAG

	Kali.phos.	6x
	Natrum sulph.	6x
	Calc.sulph.	6x

JOCK ITCH

	Natrum sulph.	6x
	Kali.sulph.	6x
	Calc.sulph.	6x

JOINTS DISEASES (See Arhtritis, Bursitis)

JUVENILE RHEUMATOID ARTHTRITIS

	Ferrum phos	6x
	Natrum sulph.	6x
	Calc.sulph.	6x

KALA AZAR (Leishmania infection)
	Kali.phos.	6x
	Natrum sulph.	6x
	Kali.sulph.	6x
	Calc.sulph.	6x

KAWASAKI DISEASE
	Kali.phos.	6x
	Natrum sulph.	6x
	Kali sulph.	6x

KELOID
1. Recent cases

	Natrum sulph.	6x
	Kali.sulph.	6x
	Silicea	6x

2. Old cases

	Kali.sulph.	6x
	Calc.sulph.	6x
	Silicea	6x

(External application: Calc.sulph. 3x, mixed in water)

KERATITIS (Inflammation of cornea)
	Ferrum phos	6x
	Natrum sulph.	6x
	Calc.sulph.	6x

KERATOCONUS
	Kali.phos.	6x
	Natrum sulph.	6x
	Kali sulph.	6x

KIDNEY DISEASES
1. Abscess (perinephritic)

	Kali.phos.	6x
	Kali.sulph.	6x
	Calc.sulph.	6x

2. Albuminuria
	Kali.mur.	6x
	Kali.sulph.	6x
	Calc.sulph.	6x
3. Anuria (no or less urine formation by kidney)
	Ferrum phos	6x
	Natrum mur.	6x
	Kali.sulph.	6x
4. Cyst in kidney
	Natrum mur.	6x
	Kali.sulph.	6x
	Calc.sulph.	6x
5. Failure - Acute renal failure (ARF)
	Natrum sulph.	6x
	Kali.sulph.	6x
	Calc.sulph.	6x
6. Failure - Chronic renal failure (CRF)
	Natrum mur.	6x
	Kali.mur.	6x
	Calc.sulph.	6x
7. Glomerular filtration rate (GFR), decreased
	Kali.sulph.	6x
	Calc.sulph.	6x
	Silicea	6x
8. Inflammation of kidney (Nephritis)
	Acute nephritis
	Kali.sulph.	6x
	Calc.sulph.	6x
	Silicea	6x
	a. Chronic nephritis with atrophy (shrinkage of kidney)
	Natrum mur.	6x
	Kali.mur.	6x
	Calc.sulph.	6x

9. With dropsy or edema
   - Kali.phos. 6x
   - Natrum mur. 6x
   - Calc.sulph. 6x
10. With symptoms of uraemia
    - Natrum mur. 6x
    - Kali.sulph. 6x
    - Calc.sulph. 6x
11. Kidney stones (Renal calculi)
    a. General remedy
       - Calc.phos. 6x
       - Natrum mur. 6x
       - Calc.sulph. 6x
    b. Calcium oxalate stones
       - Natrum sulph. 6x
       - Kali.sulph. 6x
       - Calc.sulph. 6x
    c. Phosphate stones
       - Calc.phos. 6x
       - Calc.sulph. 6x
       - Silicea 6x
    d. To eliminate the tendency of stone formation
       - Ferrum phos 6x
       - Natrum sulph. 6x
       - Calc.sulph. 6x
12. Renal colic
    a. General formula
       - Ferrum phos 6x
       - Mag.phos. 6x
       - Calc.sulph. 6x
    b. Worse, left side
       - Kali.sulph. 6x
       - Calc.sulph. 6x
       - Silicea 6x

c. Worse, right side

Kali.phos.	6x
Calc.sulph.	6x
Silicea	6x

13. Tuberculosis of kidney

Kali.sulph.	6x
Calc.sulph.	6x
Calc.flor.	6x
Silicea	6x

14. Uremia (See Uremia also)
15. Uremia-General fromula

Natrum sulph.	6x
Kali.sulph.	6x
Calc.sulph.	6x

16. Uraemic coma

Calc.phos.	6x
Kali.phos.	6x
Natrum sulph.	6x
Calc.sulph.	6x

17. Uraemic vomiting

Kali.sulph.	6x
Calc.sulph.	6x
Silicea	6x

KNEES

1. Arthritis-knee joint

Kali.sulph.	6x
Kali.mur.	6x
Natrum mur.	6x

2. Cracking sound-knee joint

Calc.sulph.	6x
Natrum sulph.	6x
Calc.flor.	6x

3. Gives way (knee can not bear the body weight)

Calc.sulph.	6x
Kali.mur.	6x
Calc.flor.	6x

4. Injuries-knee joint
　　　　　　　　　　Calc.sulph.　6x
　　　　　　　　　　Kali.mur.　　6x
　　　　　　　　　　Silicea　　　6x
5. Weakness of knee joint
　　　　　　　　　　Calc.phos.　 6x
　　　　　　　　　　Calc.sulph.　6x
　　　　　　　　　　Calc.flor.　 6x

L

LABOR (Parturition, Delivery)
1. Delayed labor-to hasten the process of delivery
   - Kali.phos. 6x
   - Natrum sulph. 6x
   - Calc.sulph. 6x

   Dose: Repeat after every 10 minutes.

2. Easy labor formula
   - Mag.phos. 6x
   - Calc.phos. 6x
   - Kali.phos. 6x
   - Calc.fluor. 6x

   Dose: once daily for first 7 months and 3 times daily during last two months of pregnancy.

3. Retention of urine or involuntary urine, after labor
   - Kali.phos. 6x
   - Kali.sulph. 6x
   - Calc.sulph. 6x

   Dose: Repeat after every 20 mnutes (total 6 doses).

4. Large abdomen, after labor
   - Nat.phos. 6x
   - Natrum sulph. 6x
   - Calc.sulph. 6x

LACRIMATION
   - Nat.phos. 6x
   - Natrum sulph. 6x
   - Calc.sulph. 6x

(See Epiphora also)

LACTATION (mother's milk) (See Breasts)

LACTATION (See Breasts)

LAGOPHTHALMOS
   - Kali.phos. 6x
   - Natrum mur. 6x
   - Calc.sulph. 6x

LARYNGITIS

Natrum sulph. 6x
Kali.sulph. 6x
Calc.sulph. 6x
Silicea 6x

LARYNGOMALACIA

Kali.phos. 6x
Natrum sulph. 6x
Calc.sulph. 6x

LASSA FEVER (Acute viral hemorrhagic illness)

Natrum mur. 6x
Kali.sulph. 6x
Calc.sulph. 6x

LEGS

1. Anterior tibial compartment syndrome (due to obstruction of venous return of blood)

   Natrum mur. 6x
   Calc.sulph. 6x
   Silicea 6x

2. Coldness of legs

   Calc.phos. 6x
   Natrum sulph. 6x
   Silicea 6x

3. Emaciation of legs (wasting of muscles)

   Kali.phos. 6x
   Kali.sulph. 6x
   Calc.sulph. 6x

4. Heaviness sensation, in legs

   Kali.phos. 6x
   Kali.sulph. 6x
   Calc.sulph. 6x

5. Intermittent claudication (pain in calf muscles on exertion)

   Kali.phos. 6x
   Natrum sulph. 6x
   Calc.sulph. 6x

6. Numbness, going asleep, neuropathies-legs
   - Kali.phos. 6x
   - Kali.sulph. 6x
   - Calc.sulph. 6x
7. Pain in calf muscles
   - Kali.sulph. 6x
   - Calc.sulph. 6x
   - Silicea 6x
8. Pain, whole legs
   - Natrum sulph. 6x
   - Calc.sulph. 6x
   - Silicea 6x
9. Cramps, contraction in leg muscles
   - Natrum sulph. 6x
   - Kali.sulph. 6x
   - Calc.sulph. 6x
10. Weak legs, difficulty in rising from a seat
    - Kali.phos. 6x
    - Natrum sulph. 6x
    - Calc.sulph. 6x

LEPROSY
- Kali.sulph. 6x
- Calc.sulph. 6x
- Silicea 6x

LEUCODERMA (Vitiligo)
- Ferrum phos 6x
- Natrum sulph. 6x
- Kali sulph. 6x

LEUKAEMIA
- Nat. Sulph 6x
- Kali.sulph. 6x
- Silicea 6x

LEUCOCYTOSIS (Excess of white blood cells in blood)
- Calc.phos. 6x
- Natrum sulph. 6x
- Calc.sulph. 6x

LEUCODERMA (See Vitiligo)

LEUCOPENIA (Deficiency of white blood cells in blood)
  Calc.phos.   6x
  Kali.phos.   6x
  Natrum sulph. 6x

LEUCORRHOEA
1. General formula
   Calc.Phos   6x
   Kali.Sulph 6x
   Calc.sulph. 6x
2. Leucorrhea-Acrid or corroding the skin
   Kali.phos. 6x
   Kali.sulph. 6x
   Calc.sulph. 6x
3. Leucorrhea-Bloody discharge
   Kali.phos.   6x
   Natrum sulph. 6x
   Calc.sulph.   6x
4. Leucorrhea-Excessive quantity, profuse
   Kali.phos. 6x
   Kali.mur.   6x
   Calc.sulph. 6x
5. Leucorrhea-Foetid, bad smelling discharge
   Kali.phos. 6x
   Kali.mur.   6x
   Calc.sulph. 6x
6. Leucorrhea-Little girls
   Kali.mur.   6x
   Kali.sulph. 6x
   Calc.sulph. 6x
7. Leucorrhea-Yellow or white disharge
   Natrum sulph. 6x
   Kali.sulph.   6x
   Calc.sulph.   6x

LICE INFESTATION (Phthrisis)
  Natrum sulph. 6x
  Calc.flor.   6x
  Silicea   6x

LICHEN

1. Lichen planus

Calc.sulph.	6x
Calc.flor.	6x
Silicea	6x

2. Lichen simplex

Natrum sulph.	6x
Kali.sulph.	6x
Silicea	6x

LIGHT-HEADEDNESS

Kali.phos.	6x
Natrum sulph.	6x
Calc.sulph.	6x

LIMB GIRDLE MUSCULAR DYSTROPHY

Kali.phos.	6x
Natrum sulph.	6x
Calc.sulph.	6x

LIPOMA

Kali.sulph.	6x
Calc.sulph.	6x
Silicea	6x

External application: Calc.flor.-3x, in water, 3 times daily.

LIPS (See Mouth, external)

LIVER DISORDERS

1. Abscess of liver

Natrum sulph.	6x
Kali.sulph.	6x
Calc.sulph.	6x

2. Cancer of liver

Natrum sulph.	6x
Kali.sulph.	6x
Calc.sulph.	6x

3. Cirrhosis (atrophy of liver) with or without ascites

Natrum sulph.	6x
Kali.sulph.	6x
Calc.sulph.	6x

Dose: 3 table 3 hourly for one week; after that 4 times daily.

4. Congestion of liver-(Acute)

Natrum sulph.	6x
Kali.mur.	6x
Calc.sulph.	6x

5. Congestion of liver-(Chronic)

Natrum sulph.	6x
Calc.sulph.	6x
Calc.flor.	6x

6. Enlargement of liver (Hypertrophy of liver)

Kali.phos.	6x
Natrum sulph.	6x
Calc.sulph.	6x

7. Failure of liver (Acute)

Ferrum phos	6x
Natrum sulph.	6x
Calc.sulph.	6x

8. Failure of liver (Chronic)

Calc.phos.	6x
Natrum sulph.	6x
Kali sulph.	6x

9. Hepatitis - A & E

Natrum sulph.	6x
Kali.sulph.	6x
Calc.sulph.	6x

10. Hepatitis - B

Kali.phos.	6x
Natrum sulph.	6x
Calc.sulph.	6x

11. Hepatitis - C

	Kali.sulph.	6x
	Calc.sulph.	6x
	Silicea	6x

12. Hepatitis-due to drugs and toxins

	Ferrum phos	6x
	Natrum sulph.	6x
	Kali sulph.	6x

LIVER SPOTS

	Ferrum phos	6x
	Natrum mur.	6x
	Natrum sulph.	6x

LOCOMOTOR ATAXIA

	Kali.mur.	6x
	Calc.sulph.	6x
	Silicea	6x

LOW BLOOD PRESSURE

	Ferrum phos.	6x
	Calc. flor.	6x
	Silicea	6x

LUMBAGO (See Backache)

LUMBAR CANAL STENOSIS (Narrowing of spinal canal)

	Natrum sulph.	6x
	Kali.sulph.	6x
	Calc.sulph.	6x

LUNGS
1. General formula

	Kali.phos.	6x
	Natrum sulph.	6x
	Calc.sulph.	6x

2. Abscess, lung

	Mag.phos.	6x
	Natrum sulph.	6x
	Calc.sulph.	6x

3. Bronchospasm

	Kali.sulph.	6x
	Calc.sulph.	6x
	Calc.flor.	6x

4. Congestion of lungs - acute

	Natrum sulph.	6x
	Kali.sulph.	6x
	Calc.sulph.	6x

5. Haemoptysis - due to tuberculosis

	Kali.sulph.	6x
	Calc.sulph.	6x
	Silicea	6x

6. Haemoptysis - due to other causes

	Kali.phos.	6x
	Kali.sulph.	6x
	Calc.sulph.	6x

7. Infiltration of lungs with eosinophils

	Ferrum phos	6x
	Kali.mur.	6x
	Calc.sulph.	6x

8. Oedema of lung (Pulmonary oedema)

	Kali.phos.	6x
	Natrum sulph.	6x
	Calc.sulph.	6x

9. Pleurisy (See Pleurisy)

10. Rattling sound with mucus

	Calc.phos.	6x
	Natrum sulph.	6x
	Calc.sulph.	6x

11. Pneumoconioses

	Natrum mur.	6x
	Natrum sulph.	6x
	Calc.sulph.	6x

12. Pneumonia (See Pneumonia)

13. Rhonchi and crepitaions in chest - (on auscultation)
 Kali.phos. 6x
 Mag.phos. 6x
 Natrum sulph. 6x

14. Silicosis
 Kali.phos. 6x
 Calc.sulph. 6x
 Silicea 6x
15. Thombosis, pulmonary
 Natrum mur. 6x
 Kali.mur. 6x
 Calc.sulph. 6x
16. Tuberculosis, pulmonary
 Natrum sulph. 6x
 Kali.sulph. 6x
 Calc.sulph. 6x

LUPUS (SLE)- Systemic lupus erythematosis
 Natrum sulph. 6x
 Kali.sulph. 6x
 Calc.sulph. 6x
LYME DISEASE
 Kali.phos. 6x
 Natrum mur. 6x
 Calc.sulph. 6x
LYMPH NODES-DISORDERS (See adenitis)

M

MALABSORPTION SYNDROME
                          Natrum sulph.   6x
                          Kali.sulph.   6x
                          Calc.sulph.   6x

MALARIA
1. Recent cases
                          Kali.phos.   6x
                          Natrum sulph.   6x
                          Calc.sulph.   6x
2. Periodical, every week, month or year
                          Calc.sulph.   6x
                          Calc.flor.   6x
                          Silicea   6x
3. Prophylactic (preventive): formula for malaria
                          Kali.phos.   12x
                          Calc.sulph.   12x
                          Silicea   12x
(one dose once a week during malaria season)

MALNUTRITION-MALNOURISHED CHILD/ADULT
                          Calc.phos.   6x
                          Kali.phos.   6x
                          Natrum sulph.   6x
                          Silicea   6x

MAMMARY GLANDS, DISEASES See Breasts

MANIA (Mental disorders with extreme anger)
                          Kali.phos.   6x
                          Kali sulph.   6x
                          Calc.sulph.   6x

MARASMUS, KWASHIORKORE (Malnutrition in children)

Calc.phos.	6x
Kali.phos.	6x
Natrum mur.	6x

(It is also good for weight loss and weakness in adults)

MASTITIS (inflammation of breast)

Kali.sulph.	6x
Calc.sulph.	6x
Silicea	6x

MASTOIDITIS (Inflammatin of mastoid)

Kali.mur.	6x
Kali.sulph.	6x
Calc.sulph.	6x

MASTURBATION
1. Ill-effects of masturbation

Calc.phos.	6x
Kali.phos.	6x
Natrum sulph.	6x

2. To quit the habit (males)

Kali.phos.	6x
Natrum mur.	6x
Kali.mur.	6x

3. To quit the habit (females)

Kali.phos.	6x
Natrum sulph.	6x
Calc.sulph.	6x

MELANCHOLIA (Severe depression)

Kali.sulph.	6x
Calc.sulph.	6x
Silicea	6x

MEASLES
1. General formula

Calc.phos.	6x
Natrum sulph.	6x
Calc.sulph.	6x

2. Measles - with cough, ear or joint pain

Kali.phos.	6x
Kali.sulph.	6x
Calc.sulph.	6x

3. Measles - with eye symptoms (inflammation) predominant
   - Kali.sulph. 6x
   - Calc.sulph. 6x
   - Silicea 6x
4. Measles - with cerebral and convulsive symptoms
   - Kali.phos. 6x
   - Kali.mur. 6x
   - Calc.sulph. 6x
5. Measles- with rash: retrocedent, or slowly developing
   - Kali.sulph. 6x
   - Calc.sulph. 6x
   - Silicea 6x

MELASMA
- Kali.sulph. 6x
- Calc.sulph. 6x
- Silicea 6x

MEMORY DISORDERS
1. Amnesia, weak, impaired memory
   - Calc.phos. 6x
   - Kali.phos. 6x
   - Calc.sulph. 6x
2. Amnesia of recent memory
   - Kali.phos. 6x
   - Natrum sulph. 6x
   - Calc.sulph. 6x
3. Difficulty of fixing attention
   - Kali.phos. 6x
   - Kali.mur. 6x
   - Silicea 6x
4. Omits, forgets letters or words while writing or talking
   - Kali.sulph. 6x
   - Calc.flor. 6x
   - Calc.sulph. 6x
5. Thoughts vanish while reading, talking, and writing
   - Kali.phos. 6x
   - Calc.phos. 6x
   - Calc.sulph. 6x

MENIERE'S DISEASE (Vertigo with tinnitus and nausea)
    Calc.sulph. 6x
    Kali.sulph. 6x
    Kali.mur. 6x

MENINGITIS
1. General formula
    Calc.sulph. 6x
    Kali.sulph. 6x
    Kali.phos. 6x
2. Bacterial meningitis
    Kali.phos. 6x
    Natrum mur. 6x
    Kali.mur. 6x
    Calc.sulph. 6x
3. Fungal meningitis
    Mag.phos. 6x
    Natrum sulph. 6x
    Kali.sulph. 6x
4. Tubercular meningitis
    Kali.sulph. 6x
    Natrum sulph. 6x
    Kali.phos. 6x
5. Viral meningitis
    Kali.phos. 6x
    Natrum sulph. 6x
    Kali.sulph. 6x
    Calc.sulph. 6x

MENOPAUSE PROBLEMS (See Climacteric for details)
1. General formula
    Kali.sulph. 6x
    Calc.sulph. 6x
    Silicea 6x

MENSTRUATION DISORDERS
1. Amenorrhoea (Stoppage of menses)
   - Kali.phos. 6x
   - Natrum sulph. 6x
   - Calc.sulph. 6x
2. Menstruation-Before expected date
   - Kali.phos. 6x
   - Calc.flor. 6x
   - Silicea 6x
3. Menstruation-Before the proper age (early menarche)
   - Kali.phos. 6x
   - Calc.sulph. 6x
   - Silicea 6x
4. Menstruation-Delayed first menses (delayed menarche)
   - Natrum mur. 6x
   - Kali.mur. 6x
   - Calc.sulph. 6x
5. Menstruation-Dysmenorrhoea (Painful menses)
   - Natrum sulph. 6x
   - Kali.mur. 6x
   - Calc.sulph. 6x
6. Menstruation-Irregular periods
   - Kali.phos. 6x
   - Natrum sulph. 6x
   - Calc.sulph. 6x
7. Menstruation-Spasmodic, with uterine congestion
   - Kali.sulph. 6x
   - Calc.sulph. 6x
   - Kali.phos. 6x
8. Menstruation-Dysmenorroea, after miscarriage or labor
   - Kali.phos. 6x
   - Calc.sulph. 6x
   - Kali sulph. 6x

9. Menstruation-Menorrhagia (menstrual periods with abnormally heavy or prolonged bleeding)
   - Kali.phos. 6x
   - Kali.sulph. 6x
   - Calc.sulph. 6x

MENSTRUATION-Complaints, preceding and during flow

1. Abdomen distended
   - Calc.sulph. 6x
   - Calc.flor. 6x
   - Silicea 6x
2. Breasts, tender, swollen
   - Kali.sulph. 6x
   - Calc.sulph. 6x
   - Silicea 6x
3. Headache
   - Kali.sulph. 6x
   - Calc.sulph. 6x
   - Silicea 6x
4. Hysterical symptoms
   - Kali.phos. 6x
   - Calc.sulph. 6x
   - Kali.mur. 6x
5. Mania, rage, anger, irritability, aggression
   - Kali.phos. 6x
   - Kali.mur. 6x
   - Calc.sulph. 6x
6. Pain labor like, goes down to hip, groins, thighs and legs
   - Calc.sulph. 6x
   - Kali.mur. 6x
   - Kali.phos. 6x
7. Pain in ovaries
   - Kali.phos. 6x
   - Natrum sulph. 6x
   - Calc.sulph. 6x

MENORRHAGIA (Menstrual periods with abnormally heavy or prolonged bleeding)
      Kali.phos. 6x
      Kali.sulph. 6x
      Calc.sulph. 6x

MENTAL DISORDERS
1. ADHD (See Attention deficit hyperactivity disorders)
2. Anxiety (See Anxiety)
3. Autism (See Autism)
4. Bipolar disorder (Period of elevated moods alternating with a phase of depression)
      Kali.phos. 6x
      Kali.mur. 6x
      Calc.flor. 6x
5. Bites himself
      Natrum sulph. 6x
      Kali.phos. 6x
      Calc.sulph. 6x
6. Delirium tremens (due to withdrawal of alcohol)
      Kali.sulph. 6x
      Calc.sulph. 6x
      Silicea 6x
7. Destructive behavior: Barks, breaks, bites, strikes
      Kali.phos. 6x
      Natrum sulph. 6x
      Calc.sulph. 6x
8. Developmental delays:
 a. Cognition (learning) delay
      Kali.phos. 6x
      Kali.sulph. 6x
      Calc.sulph. 6x
 b. Communication disorders
      Kali.phos. 6x
      Natrum mur. 6x
      Natrum sulph. 6x

c. Motor skills, delay in learing
    Kali.sulph.   6x
    Calc.sulph.   6x
    Calc.flor.   6x
d. Social functioning
    Kali.phos.   6x
    Calc.flor.   6x
    Silicea   6x
e. Speech delay
    Ferrum phos   6x
    Kali.sulph.   6x
    Calc.sulph.   6x
9. Dissociation disordes
    Ferrum phos   6x
    Natrum sulph. 6x
    Kali sulph.   6x

10. Depersonalization disorder
    Natrum sulph. 6x
    Kali.sulph.   6x
    Calc.sulph.   6x
11. Intellectual disability (mental retardation)
    Kali.phos.   6x
    Natrum sulph. 6x
    Calc.sulph.   6x
12. Lascivious mania, becomes naked
    Natrum sulph. 6x
    Kali.sulph.   6x
    Calc.sulph.   6x
13. Loquacity, talks incessantly
    Calc.phos.   6x
    Kali.sulph.   6x
    Calc.sulph.   6x
14. Panic disorder or attack
    Kali.phos.   6x
    Kali.sulph.   6x
    Silicea   6x

15. Somatic symptoms disorders
   a. Conversion disorder
Natrum mur.	6x
Kali.sulph.	6x
Calc.sulph.	6x

   b. Factitious (artificially created) disorders
Kali.phos.	6x
Natrum mur.	6x
Kali.mur.	6x

   c. Illness anxiety disorder
Natrum mur.	6x
Natrum sulph.	6x
Kali sulph.	6x

   d. Somatic symptoms disorder
Kali.mur.	6x
Kali.sulph.	6x
Calc.sulph.	6x

   (See Somatoform disorders also)

16. Stress-related disorders
   a. Adjustment disorders
Kali.sulph.	6x
Calc.sulph.	6x
Calc.flor.	6x

   b. Post-traumatic stress disorder (PTSD)
Kali.sulph.	6x
Calc.sulph.	6x
Silicea	6x

(See ADHD, Autism, Depression, Delirium, Mania, Memory, Tics, Trichotillomania, Moods, e.g., anxiety, apathetic, aversion).

METABOLIC DISORDERS

Kali.sulph.	6x
Calc.sulph.	6x
Calc.flor.	6x

METRITIS, ENDOMETRITIS (Inflammtion of uterus)
1. Acute endometritis

Kali.phos.	6x
Natrum sulph.	6x
Calc.sulph.	6x

2. Chronic endometritis

Kali.phos.	6x
Kali.mur.	6x
Calc.sulph.	6x

3. Haemorrhagic cases

Kali.sulph.	6x
Calc.sulph.	6x
Silicea	6x

METRORRHAGIA (Bleeding other than menses)

Kali.sulph.	6x
Calc.sulph.	6x
Silicea	6x

MIDDLE EAST RESPIRATORY SYNDROME (MERS)

Kali.phos.	6x
Natrum sulph.	6x
Kali.sulph.	6x
Calc.sulph.	6x

MIGRAINE
1. General formula

Kali.phos.	6x
Natrum sulph.	6x
Kali.sulph.	6x
Calc.sulph.	6x

2. Left half of head

Kali.phos.	6x
Kali.sulph.	6x
Calc.sulph.	6x
Silicea	6x

3. Right half of head
     Kali.phos. 6x
     Natrum mur. 6x
     Kali.mur. 6x

MILIARIA (Prickly heat)
     Mag.phos. 6x
     Natrum mur. 6x
     Calc.sulph. 6x

MILK (See Breasts)

MISCARRIAGE (Death of embryo before 20th week of pregnancy)
     Natrum sulph. 6x
     Kali.sulph. 6x
     Calc.sulph. 6x

MITRAL STENOSIS
     Kali.phos. 6x
     Natrum sulph. 6x
     Calc.sulph. 6x

MOODS (See Mental disorders also)
1. Anxiety(See Mental disorders also)
2. Apathetic, indifferent to everything
     Kali.phos. 6x
     Kali.sulph. 6x
     Calc.sulph. 6x
3. Aversion to physical and mental work, indecisive
     Kali.sulph. 6x
     Calc.sulph. 6x
     Calc.flor. 6x
4. Mood swings
     Kali.phos. 6x
     Kali sulph. 6x
     Calc.sulph. 6x
5. Never a smile on face
     Silicea 6x
     Kali.sulph. 6x
     Calc.sulph. 6x

6. Stubborn
                            Calc.sulph.   6x
                            Silicea   6x
                            Kali.sulph.   6x

MORNING SICKNESS (nausea, vomiting during pregnancy) (See Hyperemesis gravidarum also)
                            Natrum sulph. 6x
                            Kali.sulph.   6x
                            Calc.flor.   6x

MORPHINE (opium, heroin) ADDICTION (See Addiction)
                            Natrum sulph. 6x
                            Kali.mur.   6x
                            Calc.sulph.   6x

MORTIFICATION, from an offence (See Aggravation)
                            Kali.phos.   6x
                            Natrum sulph. 6x
                            Calc.sulph.   6x

MOTHER MILK   (See Breasts)

MOTION SICKNESS (Travel sickness-all types)
                            Kali.phos.   6x
                            Natrum sulph. 6x
                            Calc.sulph.   6x

MOUNTAIN SICKNESS (High altitude sickness)
                            Calc.phos.   6x
                            Natrum sulph. 6x
                            Kali sulph.   6x

MOUTH, INNER (oral cavity)
1. Bleeding, excessive, after tooth extraction
                            Calc.sulph.   6x
                            Calc.flor.   6x
                            Silicea   6x

2. Canker-sores (aphthous ulcers)
                            Kali.phos.   6x
                            Natrum sulph. 6x
                            Calc.sulph.   6x

3. Dryness of mouth
        Kali.phos. 6x
        Calc.sulph. 6x
        Silicea 6x
4. Glands, salivary, inflamed
        Natrum sulph. 6x
        Kali.sulph. 6x
        Calc.sulph. 6x
5. Inflammation of oral mucosa & tongue (Stomatitis)
        Kali.sulph. 6x
        Calc.sulph. 6x
        Silicea 6x
6. Inflammation, aphthous(oral thrush-candidiasis)
        Kali.mur. 6x
        Kali.sulph. 6x
        Calc.sulph. 6x
7. Inflammation, ulcers in mouth and on tongue
        Natrum sulph. 6x
        Kali.sulph. 6x
        Calc.sulph. 6x
8. Pain in mouth, from plate of teeth
        Kali.phos. 6x
        Natrum sulph. 6x
        Calc.sulph. 6x

MOUTH, EXTERNAL

1. Corners, pearly white color
        Kali.phos. 6x
        Nat.phos. 6x
        Calc.sulph. 6x
2. Cracks, ulceration
        Ferrum phos 6x
        Natrum sulph. 6x
        Calc.sulph. 6x
3. Eruptions, around mouth
        Kali.phos. 6x
        Natrum sulph. 6x
        Calc.sulph. 6x

MOUTH, LIPS

1. Black lips

Kali.phos.	6x
Natrum mur.	6x
Calc.sulph.	6x

2. Blue, cyanosed lips

Ferrum phos	6x
Natrum sulph.	6x
Calc.sulph.	6x

3. Cracks, ulcer in middle of lower lip

Calc.phos.	6x
Natrum sulph.	6x
Calc.sulph.	6x

4. Dryness of lips

Natrum sulph.	6x
Calc.sulph.	6x
Silicea	6x

5. Numbness, tingling in lips

Natrum mur.	6x
Kali.mur.	6x
Calc.sulph.	6x

6. Picks the lips untill they bleed

Kali.phos.	6x
Natrum sulph.	6x
Calc.sulph.	6x

7. Swelling of lower lip

Ferrum phos	6x
Natrum sulph.	6x
Calc.sulph.	6x

8. Swelling of upper lip

Natrum sulph.	6x
Kali.sulph.	6x
Calc.sulph.	6x

MUCUS MEMBRANES - inflammation, ulcers

Calc.phos.	6x
Natrum mur.	6x
Calc.sulph.	6x

MULTIPLE ORGAN DYSFUNCTION SYNDROME (Sepsis)

Kali.phos.	6x
Kali.sulph.	6x
Calc.sulph.	6x
Silicea	6x

MULTIPLE SCLEROSIS (Brain and spinal cord diseases leading to various problems and even disability)

Calc.phos.	6x
Kali.phos.	6x
Natrum sulph.	6x
Calc.sulph.	6x
Silicea	6x

MUMPS (Viral Parotitis)

1. General formula

Kali.sulph.	6x
Calc.sulph.	6x
Calc.flor.	6x

2. With metastasis to testes (Orchitis)

Silicea	6x
Calc.sulph.	6x
Kali sulph.	6x

3. With metastases to ovaries (Oophoritis)

Calc.sulph.	6x
Kali.sulph.	6x
Silicea	6x

MUSCAE VOLITANTES (floaters or spots before eyes)
(See Optical and Vision disorders)

MUSCLES

1. Cramps, spasms

Kali.sulph.	6x
Calc.sulph.	6x
Silicea	6x

2. Inflammation of muscles (Myositis) and pain

Ferrum phos	6x
Mag.phos.	6x
Calc.sulph.	6x

3. Loss of muscles, atrophy, wasting

Calc.phos.	6x
Kali.phos.	6x
Kali.sulph.	6x
Calc.flor.	6x

4. Pain in muscles (Myalgia)

Ferrum phos	6x
Mag.phos.	6x
Natrum mur.	6x

5. Paralysis of muscles

Kali.phos.	6x
Natrum sulph.	6x
Calc.flor.	6x

6. Soreness of muscles

Kali.sulph.	6x
Calc.sulph.	6x
Silicea	6x

7. Weakness, debility of muscles, flaccid, hanging

Kali.phos.	6x
Natrum sulph.	6x
Calc.sulph.	6x

MUSCULAR DYSTROPHY

Calc.phos.	6x
Kali.phos.	6x
Kali.sulph.	6x
Calc.flor.	6x

MUSCULAR DYSTROPHY-Limb girdle

Kali.phos.	6x
Natrum sulph.	6x
Calc.sulph.	6x

MYASTHENIA GRAVIS

Kali.phos.	6x
Calc.sulph.	6x
Kali.sulph.	6x

MYELITIS (Inflammation of spinal cord)

1. Acute myelitis

Kali.phos.	6x
Kali.sulph.	6x
Calc.sulph.	6x

2. Chronic myelitis

Natrum sulph.	6x
Kali.sulph.	6x
Calc.sulph.	6x

MYOPIA (Near-sightedness, weak distant vision)

Kali.phos.	6x
Natrum mur.	6x
Calc.sulph.	6x

MYXOEDEMA (Hypothyroidism) (See Goiter also)

Ferrum phos	6x
Natrum mur.	6x
Calc.sulph.	6x

MYXOEDEMA-Coma, Crisis

Natrum mur.	6x
Calc.sulph.	6x
Silicea	6x

N

NAEGLERIA INFECTION (Infection caused by *a parasite,* naeglaria fowleri, which leads to encephalitis and death)

Kali.phos.	6x
Natrum sulph.	6x
Kali.sulph.	6x
Calc.sulph.	6x

NAIL BITING

Kali.phos.	6x
Natrum mur.	6x
Calc.sulph.	6x

NAILS - DISEASES

1. General formula

Kali.phos.	6x
Natrum sulph.	6x
Silicea	6x

2. Atrophy of nails

Natrum mur.	6x
Kali.sulph.	6x
Calc.sulph.	6x

3. Biting the nails

Kali.phos.	6x
Natrum mur.	6x
Calc.sulph.	6x

4. Blueness, nails

Kali.sulph.	6x
Calc.sulph.	6x
Silicea	6x

(See Cyanosis also)

5. Deformed, brittle, thick

Kali.phos.	6x
Natrum sulph.	6x
Calc.sulph.	6x

6. Eruptions, around nails

Kali.phos.	6x
Calc.sulph.	6x
Silicea	6x

7. Falling off, nails

Kali.mur.	6x
Calc.sulph.	6x
Silicea	6x

8. Fungus infection-nails

Ferrum phos	6x
Kali.mur.	6x
Calc.sulph.	6x

9. Hangnails

Kali.phos.	6x
Natrum mur.	6x
Calc.flor.	6x

10. Inflammation around nails

Natrum mur.	6x
Kali.mur.	6x
Calc.sulph.	6x

11. Inflammation, of pulp or matrix of a nail

Natrum sulph.	6x
Kali.sulph.	6x
Calc.sulph.	6x

12. Ingrwoing toe nail

Kali.phos.	6x
Natrum sulph.	6x
Calc.sulph.	6x

13. Injury, to nail matrix

Natrum mur.	6x
Kali.sulph.	6x
Calc.sulph.	6x

14. Skin around nail - dry, cracked

Natrum mur.	6x
Kali.sulph.	6x
Calc.flor.	6x

15. Spots, white on nails

Natrum sulph.	6x
Kali.sulph.	6x
Silicea	6x

NAPPY RASH

Kali.phos.	6x
Natrum sulph.	6x
Calc.sulph.	6x

NARCOLEPSY

Kali.phos.	6x
Natrum sulph.	6x
Calc.sulph.	6x

NASAL POLYP

Natrum sulph.	6x
Kali.sulph.	6x
Calc.sulph.	6x

NASWAAR ABUSE

Calc. phos.	6x
Natrum mur.	6x
Calc.sulph.	6x

NAUSEA AND VOMITING

Kali.sulph.	6x
Calc.sulph.	6x
Silicea	6x

NECROSIS (Death of the cells in an organ or tissue)
1. General formula

Kali.sulph.	6x
Calc.sulph.	6x
Silicea	6x

2. Bones-necrosis

Natrum mur.	6x
Calc.sulph.	6x
Silicea	6x

3. Vertebrae - necrosis

Kali.sulph.	6x
Calc.sulph.	6x
Silicea	6x

NEONATAL JAUNDICE (See Jaundice)
NEPHRITIS (See Kidney)

NEPHROLITHIASIS (See Kidney stones)

NEPHROSCLEROSIS (Hardening of the walls of small arteries present in the kidneys)

Calc.sulph.	6x
Natrum sulph.	6x
Natrum mur.	6x

NEPHROTIC SYNDROME

Kali.sulph.	6x
Calc.sulph.	6x
Calc.flor.	6x

NERVE INJURIES

Kali.phos.	6x
Natrum mur.	6x
Calc.flor.	6x

NERVOUS WEAKNESS (See Neurasthenia)

NEURALGIA (Pain due to inflammation or nerve damage)
1. General formula

Kali.phos.	6x
Natrum sulph.	6x
Calc.sulph.	6x

2. Brachial plexus

Calc.phos.	6x
Kali.phos.	6x
Kali.mur.	6x

3. Cervico-brachial nerves
                                        Kali.phos.   6x
                                        Natrum sulph. 6x
                                        Calc.sulph.   6x

4. Cervical spondylosis
                                        Calc.phos.   6x
                                        Kali.phos.   6x
                                        Natrum mur.   6x

5. Ciliary (ciliary neuralgia with or without glaucoma)
                                        Natrum mur.   6x
                                        Kali.sulph.   6x
                                        Calc.sulph.   6x

6. Face (trigeminal neuralgia and others)
                                        Calc.phos.   6x
                                        Kali.phos.   6x
                                        Natrum sulph. 6x

7. Intercostal neuralgia, with or without cough
                                        Kali.sulph.   6x
                                        Calc.sulph.   6x
                                        Silicea   6x

8. Left side of face, neuralgia
                                        Kali.sulph.   6x
                                        Calc.sulph.   6x
                                        Silicea   6x

9. Legs, feet, neuralgia
                                        Calc.sulph.   6x
                                        Calc.flor.   6x
                                        Silicea   6x

10. Reflex neuralgia, from decayed teeth
                                        Natrum mur.   6x
                                        Kali.mur.   6x
                                        Calc.sulph.   6x

11. Penis-neuralgia

	Natrum mur.	6x
	Kali.sulph.	6x
	Silicea	6x

12. Right side of face, neuralgia

	Calc.sulph.	6x
	Calc.flor.	6x
	Silicea	6x

13. Sciatica (See Sciatica)

14. Spermatic cord neuragia

	Kali.mur.	6x
	Calc.sulph.	6x
	Silicea	6x

15. Uterine neuralgia

	Kali.sulph.	6x
	Calc.sulph.	6x
	Silicea	6x

NEURASTHENIA (Nervous prostration or weakness)

(See weakness also)

1. General formula

	Calc.phos.	6x
	Calc.flor.	6x
	Silicea	6x

2. After injury or accident

	Natrum sulph.	6x
	Kali.sulph.	6x
	Calc.sulph.	6x

3. Unable to apply mind, weak memory

	Kali.sulph.	6x
	Calc.sulph.	6x
	Silicea	6x

4. From long continued grief
- Kali.phos. 6x
- Kali.sulph. 6x
- Kali.mur. 6x

5. Hypochondriacal tendency
- Kali.phos. 6x
- Natrum sulph. 6x
- Calc.sulph. 6x

6. Old age
- Ferrum phos 6x
- Kali.phos. 6x
- Calc.sulph. 6x

7. Multiple pregnancies
- Natrum mur. 6x
- Calc.sulph. 6x
- Silicea 6x

8. Sexual excesses, from
- Kali.phos. 6x
- Natrum mur. 6x
- Calc.sulph. 6x

NEURITIS (Inflammation of a nerve)

1. General formula
- Kali.phos. 6x
- Natrum mur. 6x
- Calc.sulph. 6x

2. Diabetic patients-neuritis
- Ferrum phos 6x
- Natrum sulph. 6x
- Calc.sulph. 6x

3. In legs (anterior crural, circumflex, lesser sciatic nerves)
- Kali.phos. 6x
- Natrum sulph. 6x
- Calc.sulph. 6x

4. Retrobulbar (behind eye), with sudden loss of sight
- Kali.phos. 6x
- Natrum sulph. 6x
- Calc.sulph. 6x
- Calc.flor. 6x

NEUROFIBROMATOSIS (Tumor of nerves)
        Kali.phos. 6x
        Natrum sulph. 6x
        Calc.sulph. 6x

NEUTROPENIA (Deficiency of neutrophils in blood)
        Natrum sulph. 6x
        Calc.sulph. 6x
        Silicea 6x

NIGHT BLINDNESS
        Kali.phos. 6x
        Natrum sulph. 6x
        Calc.sulph. 6x

NIGHT - TERRORS
1. In children
        Kali.phos. 6x
        Natrum mur. 6x
        Kali.sulph. 6x
2. In adults and old age
        Kali.phos. 6x
        Natrum sulph. 6x
        Calc.sulph. 6x

NIPPLES
1. Cracks, fissures, ulcers, inflamed, sore-nipples
        Natrum mur. 6x
        Kali.sulph. 6x
        Calc.sulph. 6x
External application: Calc. flor-3x ointment.

2. Lymph nodes, inflamed, enlarged - near nipples
        Natrum sulph. 6x
        Calc.sulph. 6x
        Calc.flor. 6x

NODOSITIES, TOPHI (Uric acid deposits in the joints)
        Natrum sulph. 6x
        Calc.sulph. 6x
        Kali.mur. 6x

NOSE-EXTERNAL

1. Frackles or butterfy rash

    Natrum mur.   6x
    Kali.sulph.   6x
    Kali.mur.   6x

2. Furuncle (boil)

    Natrum sulph.   6x
    Calc.sulph.   6x
    Silicea   6x

3. Pustules (boils filled with pus)

    Kali.sulph.   6x
    Kali.mur.   6x
    Silicea   6x

4. Warts

    Natrum sulph.   6x
    Calc.sulph.   6x
    Calc.flor.   6x

5. Eczema (alae - wings of nose)

    Kali.phos.   6x
    Natrum mur.   6x
    Calc.sulph.   6x

NOSE - INTERNAL

1. Abscess, of septum

    Natrum sulph.   6x
    Kali.sulph.   6x
    Kali.mur.   6x

2. Boil, inside nose

    Natrum sulph.   6x
    Kali.sulph.   6x
    Calc.sulph.   6x

3. Caries of bone, periostitis, ulcer

    Natrum mur.   6x
    Natrum sulph.   6x
    Kali sulph.   6x

4. Deviated nasal septum (DNS)

Calc.sulph.	6x
Kali.sulph.	6x
Natrum sulph.	6x

5. Epistaxis

Ferrum phos	6x
Calc.sulph.	6x
Calc.flor.	6x

   a. With menses absent (vicarious bleeding)

Kali.phos.	6x
Kali.sulph.	6x
Calc.sulph.	6x

   b. With trauma, operations

Kali.mur.	6x
Calc.flor.	6x
Silicea	6x

6. Inflmmation (See Rhinitis)
7. Septum of nose - ulcer

Kali.phos.	6x
Kali.sulph.	6x
Calc.sulph.	6x

NOSE

1. Bad smell (See Ozaena)
2. Blowing nose - frequently

Natrum sulph.	6x
Calc.sulph.	6x
Kali.mur.	6x

3. Boring fingers, digging into nose

Natrum mur.	6x
Calc.sulph.	6x
Calc.flor.	6x

4. Congestion, obstruction – complete blockage

Kali.sulph.	6x
Calc.sulph.	6x
Silicea	6x

5. Nasal dryness

      Natrum mur. 6x
      Calc.sulph. 6x
      Calc.flor. 6x

6. Polyps in nose

      Natrum sulph. 6x
      Kali.sulph. 6x
      Calc.sulph. 6x

7. Rhinitis (inflammation of nose) (See Rhinitis)
8. Rhinosclerma (Granulomatous bacterial disease of nose)

      Natrum sulph. 6x
      Calc.sulph. 6x
      Calc.flor. 6x

9. Smell disoredrs (See Smell)

NOSTALGIA (home-sickness)

      Calc.sulph. 6x
      Calc.flor. 6x
      Silicea 6x

NUMBNESS

1. Arms - numbness

      Kali.phos. 6x
      Natrum mur. 6x
      Calc.sulph. 6x

2. Back, lumbar region - numbness

      Natrum mur. 6x
      Kali.sulph. 6x
      Kali.mur. 6x

3. Feet, hands - numbness

      Kali.phos. 6x
      Natrum mur. 6x
      Calc.sulph. 6x

4. Finger tips - numbness

      Calc.phos. 6x
      Kali.phos. 6x
      Natrum mur. 6x

5. Hands - numbness, with pain in thumb & index finger
 Kali.phos. 6x
 Natrum sulph. 6x
 Calc.sulph. 6x

NUMBNESS - CAUSES

1. Diabetic neuropathy
 Kali.phos. 6x
 Kali.sulph. 6x
 Calc.sulph. 6x
2. Hands and fingers, numbness, on grasping something
 Natrum mur. 6x
 Kali.sulph. 6x
 Calc.sulph. 6x
3. Hands, numbess in the morning
 Kali.phos. 6x
 Kali.sulph. 6x
 Kali.mur. 6x
4. Hands & Fingers numb, due to:
 a. Carpel tunnel syndrome (pinching of radial nerve)
 Kali.phos. 6x
 Calc.sulph. 6x
 Calc.flor. 6x
 b. Cervical spondylosis
 Kali.phos. 6x
 Kali.sulph. 6x
 Kali.mur. 6x
 c. Cubital tunnel syndrome
 Kali.sulph. 6x
 Calc.sulph. 6x
 Kali.mur. 6x
 d. Brachial plexus injury
 Kali.phos. 6x
 Kali.sulph. 6x
 Calc.sulph. 6x
5. Peripheral neuropathy, with pin, needle sensation
 Natrum sulph. 6x
 Kali.phos. 6x
 Calc.sulph. 6x

6. Peripheral neuropathy, with wasting of muscles
 Calc.sulph. 6x
 Natrum sulph. 6x
 Kali.phos. 6x

NUMMULAR DERMATITIS (Coin-shaped or circular spots)
 Calc.sulph. 6x
 Natrum sulph. 6x
 Kali sulph. 6x

NYMPHOMANIA (See Sex desire in females)
(See Satyriasis for uncontrollable sex desire in males also)

O

OBESITY
    Natrum mur.   6x
    Kali.sulph.   6x
    Kali.mur.   6x

OBSESSIVE COMPULSIVE DISORDER (OCD)
    Natrum sulph.   6x
    Kali.sulph.   6x
    Calc.sulph.   6x

OEDEMA
1. General formula
    Natrum mur.   6x
    Kali.sulph.   6x
    Kali.mur.   6x

2. Abdomen (Ascites)
    Kali.phos.   6x
    Natrum sulph.   6x
    Calc.sulph.   6x

3. Chest (Hydrothorax)
    Natrum mur.   6x
    Kali.sulph.   6x
    Kali.mur.   6x

4. Face
    Calc.phos.   6x
    Natrum sulph.   6x
    Calc.sulph.   6x

5. From heart disease
    Kali.phos.   6x
    Natrum mur.   6x
    Kali sulph.   6x

6. From liver disease
    Natrum sulph.   6x
    Calc.sulph.   6x
    Silicea   6x

7. Legs and feet
    Natrum sulph.   6x
    Calc.sulph.   6x
    Silicea   6x

8. Lungs (pulmonary oedema)

Kali.phos.	6x
Natrum sulph.	6x
Calc.sulph.	6x

OESOPHAGUS

1. Burning, smarting, acidity in oesophagus

Natrum sulph.	6x
Calc.sulph.	6x
Calc.flor.	6x

2. Constriction, dysphagia or difficulty in swallowing

Natrum sulph.	6x
Calc.sulph.	6x
Calc.flor.	6x

OLD AGE, DISEASES

1. General formula

Kali.phos.	6x
Natrum sulph.	6x
Kali.sulph.	6x
Calc.flor.	6x
Silicea	6x

(Do not give Silicea to pacemaker and stent patients)

2. Ageing, premature

Kali.phos.	6x
Natrum sulph.	6x
Calc.flor.	6x

3. Alzheimer's disease

Natrum mur.	6x
Kali.mur.	6x
Calc.sulph.	6x

4. Arteriosclerosis and hypertension

Kali.phos.	6x
Calc.sulph.	6x
Calc.flor.	6x

5. Arthritis, joint and muscle stiffness

    Natrum sulph.   6x
    Kali.sulph.   6x
    Calc.sulph.   6x
    Calc.flor.   6x

6. Brain atrophy

    Ferrum phos   6x
    Mag.phos.   6x
    Natrum sulph.   6x
    Silicea   6x

7. Cancer (See Cancer)

8. Constipation

    Nat.phos.   6x
    Natrum sulph.   6x
    Calc.sulph.   6x

9. Diabetes mellitus (See diabetes)

10. Degenerative diseases: Osteoarthritis, Osteoporosis, Alzheimer's diseases, etc.

    Kali.mur.   6x
    Calc.sulph.   6x
    Silicea   6x

11. Dementia

    Kali.phos.   6x
    Kali.mur.   6x
    Calc.flor.   6x

12. Heart tonic

    Kali.phos.   6x
    Natrum mur.   6x
    Calc.sulph.   6x

13. Hypertension   See Hypertension

14. Irritability and anger

    Kali.phos.   6x
    Natrum mur.   6x
    Kali.mur.   6x

15. Joint diseases (See Arthritis)

16. Memory loss or weakness

	Kali.phos.	6x
	Natrum sulph.	6x
	Kali sulph.	6x

17. Parkinsonism

a.	Mag.phos.		6x
	Kali.mur.		6x
	Natrum mur.		6x
b.	Calc.phos.		6x
	Kali.phos.		6x
	Natrum sulph.		6x

18. Prostate hypertrophy (See prostate)

19. Sexual weakness

	Kali.phos.	6x
	Natrum sulph.	6x
	Calc.sulph.	6x

20. Weakness, physical

	Calc.phos.	6x
	Natrum sulph.	6x
	Kali sulph.	6x

21. Weakness, nerves and brain

	Kali.phos.	6x
	Natrum mur.	6x
	Calc.sulph.	6x

(See Deafness, Senile decay, Dementia, Memory, Neurasthenia, Urine, Weakness also).

ONYCHOMYCOSIS (Fungal infection of nails)

	Ferrum phos	6x
	Kali.mur.	6x
	Calc.sulph.	6x

OPHTHALMIA (Inflammation of the eye)
1. Catarrhal, purulent (with pus)

Calc.sulph.	6x
Kali.sulph.	6x
Natrum sulph.	6x

2. Neonatorum (Inflammation of eyes in newborn)

Natrum sulph.	6x
Calc.flor.	6x
Natrum mur.	6x

OPIUM ADDICTION
1. Eating habit

Kali.sulph.	6x
Calc.sulph.	6x
Silicea	6x

2. Smoking habit

Kali.phos.	6x
Kali.sulph.	6x
Calc.sulph.	6x

OPTIC NERVE DISEASES
1. Atrophy of optic nerve

Calc.sulph.	6x
Kali.sulph.	6x
Natrum sulph.	6x

2. Inflammation of optic nerev (optic neuritis)

Kali.phos.	6x
Natrum sulph.	6x
Silicea	6x

OPTICAL OR VISION DISORDERS
1. Flashes, flames, stars

Kali.phos.	6x
Natrum sulph.	6x
Kali sulph.	6x

2. Halo around light

Natrum mur.	6x
Kali.mur.	6x
Calc.sulph.	6x

3. Spots, floaters (muscae volitantes)

Kali.phos.	6x
Kali.mur.	6x
Calc.sulph.	6x

ORAL LEUKOPLAKIA (white pre-cancerous spots in mouth, other than aphthae and thrush)

Natrum sulph.	6x
Kali.sulph.	6x
Calc.sulph.	6x

ORCHITIS (See Testes)

ORGASM-in female without intercourse

Kali.phos.	6x
Calc.sulph.	6x
Silicea	6x

OSTEOARTHRITIS (See Arthritis)

OSTEOCHONDROSIS (Diseases affecting the bone growth)

Natrum mur.	6x
Kali.mur.	6x
Calc.sulph.	6x

OSTEOMYELITIS (Infection of bone marrow)

Kali.phos.	6x
Calc.sulph.	6x
Calc.flor.	6x

OSTEOPENIA (Deficiency of calcium in the bones)

Natrum sulph.	6x
Kali.sulph.	6x
Calc.flor.	6x

OTALGIA (pain in ear)
1. General formula

Natrum mur.	6x
Kali.mur.	6x
Silicea	6x

2. Pulsating, throbbing pain
   - Mag.phos. 6x
   - Nat.phos. 6x
   - Natrum sulph. 6x

OTITIS MEDIA (inflammation of middle ear)
1. Catarrhal, acute
   - Ferrum phos 6x
   - Natrum sulph. 6x
   - Calc.sulph. 6x
2. Suppurative, acute (with mastoiditis)
   - Kali.phos. 6x
   - Natrum sulph. 6x
   - Kali.sulph. 6x
   - Calc.sulph. 6x
3. Chronic SOM-(Chronic suppurative otitis media)
   - Kali.phos. 6x
   - Natrum sulph. 6x
   - Kali.sulph. 6x
   - Calc.sulph. 6x
   - Silicea 6x

OTORRHOEA (ear discharge) (see discharges also)
1. Acrid discharge, corrding the skin of ear
   - Calc.sulph. 6x
   - Natrum sulph. 6x
   - Kali.sulph. 6x
2. Bland discharge, with no smell
   - Natrum sulph. 6x
   - Kali.sulph. 6x
   - Calc.sulph. 6x

3. Bloody discharge

Kali.phos.	6x
Natrum sulph.	6x
Calc.sulph.	6x

4. Foetid, bad smelling discharge

Kali.phos.	6x
Natrum sulph.	6x
Calc.sulph.	6x

5. Pus discharge

Natrum sulph.	6x
Kali.sulph.	6x
Calc.sulph.	6x

6. Watery discharge

Ferrum phos	6x
Natrum mur.	6x
Kali.mur.	6x

OVERACTIVE, IRRITABLE BLADDER

Natrum mur.	6x
Kali.mur.	6x
Calc.sulph.	6x

OVARIES - DISEASES

1. Atrophy of ovary

Kali.sulph.	6x
Calc.sulph.	6x
Silicea	6x

2. Cysts, dropsy of ovary

Kali.phos.	6x
Natrum mur.	6x
Calc.sulph.	6x

3. Hormone imbalance

Kali.phos.	6x
Natrum sulph.	6x
Calc.sulph.	6x

4. Inflammation of ovaries (Oophoritis)
   a. Acute inflammation of ovaries

Kali.sulph.	6x
Calc.sulph.	6x
Silicea	6x

   b. Chronic inflammation of ovaries

Kali.mur.	6x
Kali.sulph.	6x
Calc.sulph.	6x

5. Pain in ovary (Ovaralgia)
   General formula

Kali.sulph.	6x
Calc.sulph.	6x
Silicea	6x

6. Left ovary

Calc.sulph.	6x
Kali.sulph.	6x
Silicea	6x

7. Right ovary

Silicea	6x
Calc.sulph.	6x
Kali sulph.	6x

OVARIES, After-effects of removal of ovaries

Natrum sulph.	6x
Kali.sulph.	6x
Calc.sulph.	6x

OVULATION - ABSENT (No ovum is formed)

Ferrum phos	6x
Natrum sulph.	6x
Calc.sulph.	6x

OVUM NORMAL, BUT NOT FERTILIZED

Ferrum phos	6x
Natrum sulph.	6x
Kali.sulph.	6x
Calc.sulph.	6x

OXYGEN SATURATION-DECREASED IN BLOOD

       Kali.sulph. 6x
       Calc.sulph. 6x
       Calc.flor. 6x

OZAENA (Foul smelling nasal discharge and atrophy of nose)

       Nat.phos. 6x
       Natrum sulph. 6x
       Calc.sulph. 6x

P

PAIN
General formula
Kali.phos. 6x
Natrum sulph. 6x
Calc.sulph. 6x
(See the respective symptoms, organs and diseases)

PAIN OF CANCER
Natrum sulph. 6x
Kali.mur. 6x
Calc.sulph. 6x
(Repeat after every 15 minutes in severe pain).

PAGET'S DISEASE (Bones are not replaced by new bone tissues and thus bones become weak and deformed)
Natrum sulph. 6x
KALI.SULPH. 6x
Silicea 6x

PALATE
1. Red, swollen, inflamed
Natrum sulph. 6x
Kali.sulph. 6x
Calc.sulph. 6x

2. Ulceration, rawness of palate
Natrum sulph. 6x
Kali.mur. 6x
Calc.sulph. 6x

PALPITATION-HEART
Calc.sulph. 6x
Calc.flor. 6x
Silicea 6x
(See Heart also)

PANARITIUM (inflammation aound a finger nail)
Kali.mur.	6x
Kali.sulph.	6x
Calc.sulph.	6x

External application: Calc.sulph.3x ointment.
(See Nail inflammation also).

PANCREAS - DISEASES
1. Acute pancreatitis, with diarrhea, vomiting and burning pain in region of pancreas
Kali.sulph.	6x
Calc.sulph.	6x
Silicea	6x

(Repeat at half hourly intervals, till improvement occurs)

2. Chronic pancreatitis
Kali.phos.	6x
Natrum sulph.	6x
Kali.sulph.	6x
Calc.sulph.	6x

3. Pancreatitis with disturbed insulin production
Natrum sulph.	6x
Kali.sulph.	6x
Calc.sulph.	6x

PANIC ATTACK (See Mental disorders also)
Kali.phos.	6x
Kali.sulph.	6x
Silicea	6x

PARA - INFLUENZA VIRUS
Natrum sulph.	6x
Kali.sulph.	6x
Calc.sulph.	6x

PARALYSIS (See Gait disorders also)
1. Arm or hand-paralysis
Kali.phos.	6x
Natrum mur.	6x
Calc.sulph.	6x

2. Hemiplegia Left (paralysis of left half of body)
   - Ferrum phos 6x
   - Natrum mur. 6x
   - Kali.mur. 6x
3. Hemiplegia, Right (paralysis of right half of body)
   - Kali.phos. 6x
   - Kali.mur. 6x
   - Calc.sulph. 6x
4. Infantile paralysis (Poliomyelitis)
   - Natrum mur. 6x
   - Natrum sulph. 6x
   - Calc.sulph. 6x
5. Paraplegia (paralysis of lower half of body or legs)
   - Kali.phos. 6x
   - Natrum sulph. 6x
   - Calc.sulph. 6x
6. Pneumogastric paralysis (paralysis of lungs)
   - Natrum sulph. 6x
   - Kali.phos. 6x
   - Kali.sulph. 6x
   - Calc.sulph. 6x
7. Forearm paralysis (Wrist-drop: paralysis of forearm and wrist)
   - Kali.phos. 6x
   - Natrum sulph. 6x
   - Kali.sulph. 6x
   - Calc.sulph. 6x
8. Sphinctres(urninary and anal sphincter paralysis)
   - Kali.phos. 6x
   - Calc.sulph. 6x
   - Natrum sulph. 6x
   - Kali.sulph. 6x
9. Throat, vocal cords-paralysis (loss of voice)
   - Calc.sulph. 6x
   - Kali.phos. 6x
   - Natrum sulph. 6x
   - Kali.sulph. 6x

PARKINSONISM (Paralysis agitans)
        Kali.phos. 6x
        Natrum sulph. 6x
        Calc.sulph. 6x
PAROTITIS (Inflammation of parotid glands by pathogens, other than mumps virus)
        Ferrum phos 6x
        Natrum mur. 6x
        Kali.sulph. 6x
        Calc.sulph. 6x

PAWN ABUSE
        Kali.phos. 6x
        Kali.sulph. 6x
        Calc.sulph. 6x

PELVIC DISEASES
1. Abscess, pelvic, pelvic inflammatory disease (PID)
        Kali.sulph. 6x
        Calc.sulph. 6x
        Calc.flor. 6x
        Silicea 6x
2. Peritonitis (inflammation of the peritoneum)
        Kali.phos. 6x
        Kali.sulph. 6x
        Calc.sulph. 6x
        Silicea 6x
3. Fallopian tubes (See Fallopian tubes)
  Ovaries   (See Ovaries)

PEMPHIGUS (Blisters on all of the skin and mucosa; an autoimmune disease)
        Natrum sulph. 6x
        Kali.sulph. 6x
        Calc.sulph. 6x

PENIS – DISORDERS (See Sexual disorders also)
1. Atrophy, small in size (children and adults)
   - Calc.sulph. 6x
   - Kali.phos. 6x
   - Natrum sulph. 6x
2. Erectile dysfunction (weak erection or fails on coition)
   - Natrum sulph. 6x
   - Kali.phos. 6x
   - Calc.sulph. 6x
3. Pain in penis
   - Natrum sulph. 6x
   - Kali.sulph. 6x
   - Calc.sulph. 6x
4. Peyronie's disease (severe deformity of penis)
   - Kali.phos. 6x
   - Natrum sulph. 6x
   - Kali.sulph. 6x
   - Calc.sulph. 6x
5. Priapism (painful erection of penis)
   - Ferrum phos 6x
   - Natrum sulph. 6x
   - Calc.sulph. 6x
6. Pustules on penis
   - Calc.sulph. 6x
   - Calc.flor. 6x
   - Silicea 6x
7. Rash and spots on penis
   - Kali.phos. 6x
   - Natrum sulph. 6x
   - Calc.sulph. 6x
8. Swollen, inflamed glans penis
   - Kali.sulph. 6x
   - Calc.sulph. 6x
   - Silicea 6x

9. Warts, condylomata (any type) on penis

  Natrum sulph. 6x
  Kali.sulph. 6x
  Calc.sulph. 6x
  Silicea 6x

PEPTIC ESOPHAGITIS (See GERD)

PEPTIC ULCER

  Kali.phos. 6x
  Natrum sulph. 6x
  Calc.sulph. 6x

PERICARDITIS (Inflammation of the pericardium, a sac covering the heart). (See Heart also)

  Natrum sulph. 6x
  Kali.sulph. 6x
  Calc.sulph. 6x

PERI-ORAL DERMATITIS

  Natrum sulph. 6x
  Kali.sulph. 6x
  Calc.sulph. 6x

PERIOSTITIS, and periosteal dieases (See Bones)

PERIPHERAL ARTERIAL DISEASES

  Kali.phos. 6x
  Natrum sulph. 6x
  Kali.sulph. 6x
  Calc.sulph. 6x

PERITONITIS

1. Acute peritonitis

  Kali.phos. 6x
  Kali.sulph. 6x
  Calc.sulph. 6x
  Silicea 6x

2. Chronic peritonitis

Kali.phos.	6x
Natrum sulph.	6x
Calc.sulph.	6x
Silicea	6x

PERTUSSIS (Whooping cough)

Kali.phos.	6x
Natrum sulph.	6x
Calc.sulph.	6x

PETECHIAE (Bleeding spots under skin)

Natrum sulph.	6x
Kali.sulph.	6x
Calc.sulph.	6x

PHTHRIASIS (Lice)

Kali.sulph.	6x
Calc.sulph.	6x
Silicea	6x

PETIT MAL EPILEPSY (See Epilepsy)

PEYRONIE'S DISEASE (Severe deformity of penis)

Kali.phos.	6x
Natrum sulph.	6x
Kali.sulph.	6x
Calc.sulph.	6x

PHARYNGITIS (inflammation of pharynx)
1. General fromula

Kali.sulph.	6x
Calc.sulph.	6x
Calc.flor.	6x

2. Catarrhal pharyngitis, acute or chronic

Kali.phos.	6x
Kali.sulph.	6x
Calc.sulph.	6x
Silicea	6x

PHLEBITIS (inflammation of vein)

Kali.sulph.	6x
Calc.sulph.	6x
Silicea	6x

PHLEGMASIA ALBA DOLENS (Milk-leg, after delivery)
  Natrum sulph. 6x
  Kali.sulph. 6x
  Calc.sulph. 6x

PHOBIAS (Fears)
1. Animals-fear
   Kali.phos. 6x
   Natrum sulph. 6x
   Calc.sulph. 6x
2. Closed spaces-fear
   Kali.phos. 6x
   Kali.sulph. 6x
   Calc.flor. 6x
3. Crowds, crossing streets-fear
   Kali.phos. 6x
   Kali.sulph. 6x
   Calc.flor. 6x
4. Examination-fear
   Kali.sulph. 6x
   Calc.sulph. 6x
   Calc.flor. 6x
5. Heights-fear
   Kali.phos. 6x
   Kali.mur. 6x
   Calc.sulph. 6x
6. Insects-fear
   Kali.mur. 6x
   Calc.sulph. 6x
   Silicea 6x
7. People-fear (Anthropophobia)
   Kali.phos. 6x
   Kali.mur. 6x
   Calc.flor. 6x

8. Solitude, (fear of loneliness)
Kali.phos.	6x
Calc.sulph.	6x
Silicea	6x

9. Stage-fright
Kali.sulph.	6x
Calc.sulph.	6x
Silicea	6x

PHOSPHATURIA (See Urine)

PHOTOPHOBIA
Kali.phos.	6x
Kali.mur.	6x
Calc.sulph.	6x

PHTHISIS (Wasting diseases, like tuberculsos, diabetes mellitus, hyperthyroidism and marasmus)
Natrum sulph.	6x
Kali.sulph.	6x
Calc.sulph.	6x

PHTHISIS, pulmonalis (wasting of lungs) See Tuberculosis

PICA (morbid appetite) (See Appetite)
PILES (See Hemorrhoids)
PILONIDAL ABSCESS, SINUS, CYST
Kali.phos.	6x
Kali.mur.	6x
Calc.sulph.	6x

PITYRIASIS VERSICOLOR (Fungal infection of skin with discolored spots)
Kali.phos.	6x
Calc.sulph.	6x
Silicea	6x

PLAGUE
Kali.phos.	6x
Natrum sulph.	6x
Calc.sulph.	6x

PLEURISY
1. General formula

	Kali.sulph.	6x
	Calc.sulph.	6x
	Silicea	6x

2. With adhesions

	Kali.sulph.	6x
	Calc.sulph.	6x
	Calc.flor.	6x

3. With cancer of lungs

	Kali.phos.	6x
	Kali.sulph.	6x
	Calc.sulph.	6x

4. With pleural effusion

	Kali.phos.	6x
	Natrum sulph.	6x
	Silicea	6x

5. With tuberculosis

	Kali.sulph.	6x
	Calc.sulph.	6x
	Silicea	6x

PLEURITIS

	Natrum sulph.	6x
	Kali.sulph.	6x
	Calc.sulph.	6x

PMS (See Pre-menstrual syndrome)
PNEUMONIA (Broncho-pneumonia)

	Kali.phos.	6x
	Kali.mur.	6x
	Calc.sulph.	6x

POISONING
1. By mouth, poison

	Kali.phos.	6x
	Natrum sulph.	6x
	Calc.sulph.	6x

2. Carbon monoxide or sewer gas poisoning by inhalation

Natrum sulph.	6x
Kali.sulph.	6x
Calc.sulph.	6x

Dose: Repeat after every ten minutes in both cases.

3. Food poisoning   (See Food poisoning)

POLIOMYELITIS   (See Paralysis, infantile)

POLYCHROME SPECTRA, optical illusions

1. Black spots before eyes

Kali.sulph.	6x
Calc.sulph.	6x
Silicea	6x

2. Flashes, flames, flickering

Kali.phos.	6x
Natrum mur.	6x
Kali sulph.	6x

3. Halo around light

Natrum mur.	6x
Kali.mur.	6x
Calc.sulph.	6x

4. Sparks, stars

Kali.phos.	6x
Natrum sulph.	6x
Calc.sulph.	6x

5. Spots, floaters (muscae volitantes)

Kali.sulph.	6x
Calc.sulph.	6x
Calc.flor.	6x

POLYCYSTIC OVARIAN DISEASE

1. General formula

Kali.phos.	6x
Natrum mur.	6x
Calc.sulph.	6x

2. Absent or scanty menses

Kali.phos.	6x
Kali.sulph.	6x
Calc.flor.	6x

3. Cysts in ovaries

Mag.phos.	6x
Nat.phos.	6x
Calc.sulph.	6x

4. Hair on face in femlaes

Kali.phos.	6x
Kali.mur.	6x
Calc.sulph.	6x

5. Hormone imbalance

Kali.phos.	6x
Calc.sulph.	6x
Silicea	6x

6. Impaired blood glucose levels

Natrum mur.	6x
Natrum sulph.	6x
Calc.sulph.	6x

7. Irregular periods

Kali.phos.	6x
Kali.sulph.	6x
Calc.sulph.	6x

8. Obesity

Calc.sulph.	6x
Calc.flor.	6x
Silicea	6x

9. Prolonged menses

Ferrum phos	6x
Natrum sulph.	6x
Kali sulph.	6x

10. Excessive male hormone, in women

Kali.sulph.	6x
Calc.sulph.	6x
Silicea	6x

POLYMYALGIA RHEUMATICA

Kali.phos. 6x
Natrum sulph. 6x
Calc.sulph. 6x
Silicea 6x

POLYNEUROPATHY

Kali.sulph. 6x
Calc.sulph. 6x
Silicea 6x

POLYPS

1. All types

Kali.sulph. 6x
Calc.sulph. 6x
Calc.flor. 6x

2. Colon, polyp

Calc.sulph. 6x
Calc.flor. 6x
Silicea 6x

3. Gall bladder, polyp

Calc.sulph. 6x
Calc.flor. 6x
Silicea 6x

4. Nose, polyp

Ferrum phos 6x
Natrum sulph. 6x
Calc.sulph. 6x

5. Rectal, polyp

Calc.sulph. 6x
Calc.flor. 6x
Silicea 6x

6. Uterus, polyps

Kali.sulph. 6x
Calc.sulph. 6x
Silicea 6x

POLYURIA

Kali.phos.	6x
Natrum sulph.	6x
Calc.sulph.	6x

PORTAL HYPERTENSION

Calc.sulph.	6x
Kali.sulph.	6x
Silicea	6x

POST- NASAL DISEASES (naso-pharynx)

1. Inflammation, acute

Natrum mur.	6x
Kali.mur.	6x
Calc.sulph.	6x

2. Inflammation, chronic

Kali.sulph.	6x
Calc.sulph.	6x
Silicea	6x

3. Inflammation, chronic, with post-nasal dropping

Kali.mur.	6x
Calc.sulph.	6x
Silicea	6x

POST-TRAUMATIC STRESS DISORDER (PTSD)

Kali.sulph.	6x
Calc.sulph.	6x
Silicea	6x

PRECOCIOUS PUBERTY (males)

Kali.phos.	6x
Natrum sulph.	6x
Calc.sulph.	6x

PRE - ECLAMPSIA (Toxemia of pregnancy)

Calc.phos.	6x
Calc.sulph.	6x
Silicea	6x

(See Eclampsia also)

PREGNANCY, DISORDERS

1. Albuminuria in pregnancy
   - Kali.phos. 6x
   - Natrum sulph. 6x
   - Calc.sulph. 6x
2. Anemia in pregnancy
   - Calc.phos. 6x
   - Natrum mur. 6x
   - Kali.phos. 6x
3. Backache in pregnancy
   - Calc.phos. 6x
   - Kali.phos. 6x
   - Mag.phos. 6x
4. Breasts painful, in pregnancy
   - Calc.phos. 6x
   - Kali.sulph. 6x
   - Calc.sulph. 6x
5. Constipation in pregnancy
   - Natrum mur. 6x
   - Kali.mur. 6x
   - Calc.flor. 6x
6. Cough in pregnancy
   - Calc.sulph. 6x
   - Kali.sulph. 6x
   - Silicea 6x
7. Cramps, calf muscles, in pregnancy
   - Ferrum phos 6x
   - Mag.phos. 6x
   - Natrum mur. 6x
8. Cravings, abnormal appetite (See Appetite)
9. Diabetes durin pregnance (See Diabetes-gestational)
10. Diarrhoea in pregnancy
    - Kali.phos. 6x
    - Natrum sulph. 6x
    - Calc.sulph. 6x

11. Fetus
   a. Heart beat, stops or missing beats
       - Kali.sulph. 6x
       - Calc.sulph. 6x
       - Silicea 6x
   b. Malposition or malpresentation of fetus
       - Kali.phos. 6x
       - Kali.mur. 6x
       - Calc.flor. 6x
   c. Painful movements of fetus
       - Kali.phos. 6x
       - Natrum sulph. 6x
       - Calc.sulph. 6x
   d. Slow growth of fetus
       - Calc.phos. 6x
       - Natrum sulph. 6x
       - Calc.flor. 6x

12. Morning sickness (nausea, vomiting)
    - Calc.phos. 6x
    - Kali.phos. 6x
    - Nat.phos. 6x

13. Oedema – feet, legs
    - Ferrum phos 6x
    - Natrum mur. 6x
    - Calc.sulph. 6x

14. Palpitataion during pregnancy
    - Kali.phos. 6x
    - Natrum mur. 6x
    - Silicea 6x

15. Pica (eating chalk, clay, wood, etc)
    - Calc.phos. 6x
    - Ferrum phos 6x
    - Natrum mur. 6x

16. Pruritus-vulva and vagina
- Kali.phos. 6x
- Natrum sulph. 6x
- Calc.sulph. 6x

17. Salivation-increased
- Natrum mur. 6x
- Calc.sulph. 6x
- Nat.phos. 6x

18. Sexual excitement (See Nymhomania also)
- Natrum sulph. 6x
- Kali.sulph. 6x
- Calc.flor. 6x

19. Sleeplessness during pregnancy
- Ferrum phos 6x
- Natrum sulph. 6x
- Kali sulph. 6x

20. Toothache during pregnancy
- Ferrum phos 6x
- Calc.sulph. 6x
- Silicea 6x

21. Toxaemia of pregnancy
- Ferrum phos 6x
- Natrum sulph. 6x
- Calc.sulph. 6x

22. Urinary tract infection, during prgnancy
- Kali.phos. 6x
- Nat.phos. 6x
- Calc.sulph. 6x

23. Varicose veins during pregnancy
- Calc.phos. 6x
- Calc.sulph. 6x
- Calc.flor. 6x

24. Vertigo during pragnancy
- Natrum sulph. 6x
- Calc.sulph. 6x
- Silicea 6x

25. Weakness during pragnancy
- Calc.phos. 6x
- Kali.phos. 6x
- Natrum sulph. 6x

PREMATURE EJACULATION (See Sexual disorders)

PREAMTURE GREYING OF HAIR (See Hair)

PRIAPISM (Prolonged and painful erection of the penis)
- Ferrum phos 6x
- Natrum sulph. 6x
- Calc.sulph. 6x

PRICKLY HEAT
- Mag.phos. 6x
- Natrum mur. 6x
- Calc.sulph. 6x

PROCTITIS (inflammation of the rectum and anus)
- Ferrum phos 6x
- Natrum sulph. 6x
- Calc.sulph. 6x

External application: Calc.sulph. 3x in vaseline ointment.

PROLAPSE OF ANUS
- Natrum mur. 6x
- Kali.mur. 6x
- Calc.sulph. 6x

PROLAPSE OF UTERUS

Natrum sulph. 6x
Kali.sulph. 6x
Calc.sulph. 6x
Calc.flor. 6x

PROLAPSE OF RECTUM

Kali.sulph. 6x
Calc.sulph. 6x
Calc.flor. 6x
Sil 6x

PROLAPSE OF VAGINA

Calc.phos. 6x
Kali.phos. 6x
Natrum sulph. 6x
Kali.mur. 6x

PROSOPALGIA (face-ache, neuralgia) See Neuralgia

PROSTATE GLAND DISORDERS

1. General remedy

    Calc.phos. 6x
    Kali.phos. 6x
    Natrum sulph. 6x
    Calc.sulph. 6x

2. Cancer, prostate

    Kali.phos. 6x
    Natrum sulph. 6x
    Calc.sulph. 6x

3. Hypertrophy (Benign prostate hypertrophy-BPH)

    Kali.phos. 6x
    Natrum mur. 6x
    Kali.mur. 6x
    Calc.sulph. 6x

PROSTATE, Inflammation (prostatitis)
1. Acute prostatitis
   - Kali.sulph. 6x
   - Calc.sulph. 6x
   - Silicea 6x
2. Chronic prostatitis
   - Natrum sulph. 6x
   - Kali.sulph. 6x
   - Calc.sulph. 6x

PRURITUS, ITCHING, DERMATITIS, ECZEMA
1. General remedy
   - Kali.mur. 6x
   - Kali.sulph. 6x
   - Calc.sulph. 6x
2. Of genitals
   - Kali.phos. 6x
   - Natrum sulph. 6x
   - Calc.sulph. 6x
3. Of webs of fingers, bends of joints
   - Kali.sulph. 6x
   - Calc.sulph. 6x
   - Silicea 6x
4. Amelioration from cold
   - Kali.sulph. 6x
   - Calc.sulph. 6x
   - Calc.flor. 6x
5. Amelioration from warmth
   - Natrum sulph. 6x
   - Kali.sulph. 6x
   - Calc.sulph. 6x
6. Worse from undressing, warmth of bed
   - Natrum mur. 6x
   - Kali.mur. 6x
   - Calc.sulph. 6x

PSORIASIS
	Kali.phos.	6x
	Natrum sulph.	6x
	Calc.sulph.	6x

PSORIATIC ARHTRITIS
	Natrum sulph.	6x
	Kali.sulph.	6x
	Calc.sulph.	6x

PSYCHOLOGICAL DISORDERS
(See Autism, ADHD, Depression, Mania, Memory, Mental disorders, Delirium, Moods, eg. anxiety, apathetic, aversion)

PTERYGIUM - EYE
	Ferrum phos	6x
	Natrum sulph.	6x
	Calc.flor.	6x

PTYALISM (excessive saliva)
	Natrum mur.	6x
	Kali.mur.	6x
	Calc.sulph.	6x

PUERPERAL PSYCHOSIS (Post-partum psychosis)
(A severe mental illness after delivery).
	Kali.sulph.	6x
	Calc.sulph.	6x
	Silicea	6x

PULMONARY DISEASES (Lungs diseases)
1. Congestion of lungs
	Natrum mur.	6x
	Kali sulph.	6x
	Calc.sulph.	6x

2. Edema of lungs
	Kali.phos.	6x
	Natrum sulph.	6x
	Calc.sulph.	6x

3. Embolism in lungs
	Kali.phos.	6x
	Natrum sulph.	6x
	Calc.sulph.	6x

4. Eosinophilia-pulmonary
   - Ferrum phos 6x
   - Kali.mur. 6x
   - Calc.sulph. 6x
5. Pulmonary hypertension
   - Natrum sulph. 6x
   - Kali.sulph. 6x
   - Calc.sulph. 6x

PUERPERIUM (six weeks period after childbirth)
1. Pain, lower abdomen, groins, shins
   - Kali.phos. 6x
   - Natrum sulph. 6x
   - Kali.sulph. 6x
   - Calc.sulph. 6x
2. Haemorrhage, from uterus
   - Kali.phos. 6x
   - Natrum sulph. 6x
   - Calc.sulph. 6x
3. Haemorrhoids, piles
   - Kali.phos. 6x
   - Kali.sulph. 6x
   - Calc.sulph. 6x
4. Lochia, acrid, bloody; scanty or offensive
   - Kali.phos. 6x
   - Natrum sulph. 6x
   - Kali sulph. 6x
5. Fever (milk-fever)
   - Kali.mur. 6x
   - Kali.sulph. 6x
   - Calc.sulph. 6x
6. Mania (Puerperal psychosis)
   - Kali.sulph. 6x
   - Calc.sulph. 6x
   - Silicea 6x

PULSE

1. Full, round, bounding, strong, felt all over body
   - Kali.phos. 6x
   - Kali.mur. 6x
   - Calc.sulph. 6x
2. Intermittent pulse, missing beats
   - Natrum mur. 6x
   - Kali.mur. 6x
   - Calc.sulph. 6x
3. Irregular pulse
   - Kali.phos. 6x
   - Natrum sulph. 6x
   - Calc.sulph. 6x
4. Rapid pulse (Tachycardia)
   - Kali.phos. 6x
   - Natrum sulph. 6x
   - Calc.sulph. 6x
5. Slow pulse (Bradycardia)
   - Kali.phos. 6x
   - Kali.sulph. 6x
   - Calc.sulph. 6x
6. Weak, hardly perceptible pulse
   - Kali.phos. 6x
   - Kali.sulph. 6x
   - Silicea 6x

PUNCTURED WOUNDS

- Kali.phos. 6x
- Natrum sulph. 6x
- Calc.sulph. 6x

PUPILS (See Eyes)

PURPURA (Purple spots under skin due to bursting of small blood vessels)

- Kali.mur. 6x
- Kali.sulph. 6x
- Calc.sulph. 6x

PYELITIS (Inflammation of pelvis of kidney)
1. Acute pyelitis

    Natrum sulph.   6x
    Kali.sulph.   6x
    Calc.sulph.   6x

2. Calculous, pyelitis- with kidney stone

    Kali.phos.   6x
    Kali.mur.   6x
    Calc.flor.   6x

3. Chronic pyelitis

    Calc.phos.   6x
    Natrum sulph.   6x
    Kali.mur.   6x

PYEMIA, Septicemia (bacteria and pus circulating in blood)

    Kali.sulph.   6x
    Calc.sulph.   6x
    Silicea   6x

PYLORUS (First part of small intestine which connects the stomach with duodenum)
1. Constriction of pylorus

    Calc.sulph.   6x
    Natrum sulph.   6x
    Kali.sulph.   6x

2. Pain in pylorus

    Kali.phos.   6x
    Natrum sulph.   6x
    Calc.sulph.   6x

PYORRHOEA, ALVEOLARIS (infection of alveolar socket)

    Kali.sulph.   6x
    Calc.sulph.   6x
    Silicea   6x

PYROSIS (heartburn)

Natrum sulph.	6x
Kali.sulph.	6x
Calc.sulph.	6x

PYURIA (pus cells in urine)

Kali.sulph.	6x
Calc.sulph.	6x
Silicea	6x

Q FEVER (Bacterial disease caused by Coxiella burnetii present in placenta, in Amniotic fluid, feces, urine and milk of goat, sheep and cattle).

Natrum sulph.	6x
Kali.sulph.	6x
Calc.sulph.	6x

R

RAYNAUD'S DISEASE (Spasm of blood vessels which causes decreased blood circulation to fingers, toes, knees, ears, nipples and nose)

Kali.phos.	6x
Natrum sulph.	6x
Calc.sulph.	6x

RECTUM

1. Abscess (Peri-rectal abscess)

Kali.phos.	6x
Natrum sulph.	6x
Calc.sulph.	6x
Silicea	6x

2. Burning in rectum

Natrum sulph.	6x
Kali.sulph.	6x
Calc.sulph.	6x

3. Cancer, rectum

Kali.phos.	6x
Natrum sulph.	6x
Kali.sulph.	6x
Calc.sulph.	6x

4. Paretic conditions (paralysis of rectum)

Kali.phos.	6x
Natrum sulph.	6x
Calc.sulph.	6x

5. Proctitis (inflammation of rectum)

Ferrum phos	6x
Natrum sulph.	6x
Calc.sulph.	6x

External application: Calc.sulph.- 3x ointment.

6. Prolapse of rectum
	Kali.sulph.	6x
	Calc.sulph.	6x
	Calc.flor.	6x
	Sil	6x

RENAL COLIC (See Kidney diseases and Colic)

RESTLESS LEG SYNDROME
Kali.phos.	6x
Natrum sulph.	6x
Calc.sulph.	6x

RESTLESSNESS
Calc.phos.	6x
Kali.phos.	6x
Natrum sulph.	6x

RETINA
1. Apoplexy (haemorrhage) in retina
Kali.sulph.	6x
Calc.sulph.	6x
Calc.flor.	6x

2. Congestion of retina
Calc.sulph.	6x
Kali.phos.	6x
Kali.sulph.	6x

3. Damage by lookin at welding arc light or sun rays
Kali.phos.	6x
Natrum sulph.	6x
Calc.sulph.	6x

4. Degeneration of retina
Kali.phos.	6x
Kali.sulph.	6x
Calc.sulph.	6x

5. Detachment of retina

Kali.phos.	6x
Kali.sulph.	6x
Calc.sulph.	6x

6. Hard exudate in retina

Kali.sulph.	6x
Calc.sulph.	6x
Silicea	6x

7. Injury of retina

Kali.phos.	6x
Natrum sulph.	6x
Calc.sulph.	6x

8. Soft exudate in retina

Natrum sulph.	6x
Kali.sulph.	6x
Calc.sulph.	6x

9. Thrombosis of retinal vessles

Calc.sulph.	6x
Natrum sulph.	6x
Kali.sulph.	6x

RHABDOMYOLYSIS (Breakdown of skeletal muscle fibers)

Kali.phos.	6x
Natrum sulph.	6x
Kali.sulph.	6x
Calc.sulph.	6x

RHEUMATIC FEVER

Kali.sulph.	6x
Calc.sulph.	6x
Calc.flor.	6x

RHEUMATIC HEART DISEASE

Kali.sulph.	6x
Calc.sulph.	6x
Silicea	6x

RHEUMATISM (See Arthritis)

RHINO VIRUS, INFECTIONS (Common cold, sinus infection, pneumonia and bronchiolitis caused by rhinoviruses)
        Natrum sulph. 6x
        Kali.sulph. 6x
        Calc.sulph. 6x
        Silicea 6x

RHINITIS (Inflammation of nasal mucosa with obstruction, itching in nose, runny nose, post-nasal drip and sneezing).

1. Acute rhinitis (allergic or bacterial) and Hay fever
        Kali.phos. 6x
        Natrum mur. 6x
        Kali.sulph. 6x
        Calc.sulph. 6x

2. Acute (viral) rhinitis
        Kali.phos. 6x
        Natrum sulph. 6x
        Kali.sulph. 6x
        Calc.sulph. 6x

3. Chronic rhinitis
        Kali.sulph. 6x
        Calc.sulph. 6x
        Silicea 6x

4. Predisposition or tendency to rhinitis
        Kali.phos. 6x
        Natrum sulph. 6x
        Calc.sulph. 6x

5. Coryza, worse in warm room, better in open air
        Kali.phos. 6x
        Natrum sulph. 6x
        Calc.sulph. 6x

6. Coryza, worse in open air, better in room
        Calc.sulph. 6x
        Kali.ulph. 6x
        Natrum sulph. 6x

7. Coryza, with lachrymation, sneezing
   Kali.sulph. 6x
   Calc.sulph. 6x
   Silicea 6x
8. Coryza, purulent (pus), especially in children
   Kali.phos. 6x
   Kali.sulph. 6x
   Calc.sulph. 6x

RICKETS (faulty bone development in children, leading to weak bones causing bone deformities. Disease of soft bones in adults is called osteomalacia).
   Calc.sulph. 6x
   Calc.flor. 6x
   Silicea 6x

RINGWORM (Dermatophytosis) (Fungal infection of skin)
   Ferrum phos 6x
   Nat.phos. 6x
   Natrum sulph. 6x

ROTA VIRUS DISEASE (The most common cause of severe diarrhea in children; virus is transmitted from stool of infected hands of children, toys and infected door knobs).
   Natrum sulph. 6x
   Kali.sulph. 6x
   Calc.sulph. 6x
   Silicea 6x

RUBELLA (German measles) (Viral infection in mother damage the fetus if it occurs during pregnancy).
   Natrum sulph. 6x
   Kali.mur. 6x
   Calc.sulph. 6x

Prevention of Rubella
   Natrum sulph. 6x
   Kali.sulph. 6x
   Calc.sulph. 6x

Dose: once daily, for two weeks, to girls or females before pregnancy.

S

SALPINGITIS (inflammation of fallopian tubes)
                                       Kali.sulph.   6x
                                       Calc.sulph.   6x
                                       Calc.flor.   6x

SARCOIDOSIS (Granulomas-red and swollen tissues develop in skin and lungs)
                                       Kali.sulph.   6x
                                       Calc.sulph.   6x
                                       Silicea   6x

SATYRIASIS (See Sex desire in males)

SCABIES (Severe itching and rash in skin, caused by itch mite named sarcoptes scabiei).
                                       Calc.sulph.   6x
                                       Natrum sulph.   6x
                                       Silicea   6x

External application: Calc.sulph. 3x mixed in water, 3 times daily.
Ratio: 2 ml tincture or 20 grams of tablets in 200ml of water.

SCALP DISEASES
    1. Boils, pustules, on scalp
                                     Calc.phos.   6x
                                     Kali.sulph.   6x
                                     Calc.sulph.   6x

    2. Crusta lactea, scalp
                                     Kali.sulph.   6x
                                     Calc.sulph.   6x
                                     Calc.flor.   6x

    3. Dandruff, scalp
                                     Natrum mur.   6x
                                     Kali.mur.   6x
                                     Calc.sulph.   6x

4. Eczema, scalp
- Kali.sulph. 6x
- Calc.sulph. 6x
- Silicea 6x

5. Growths, tumors, exostoses, nodes, on scalp
- Calc.flor. 6x
- Calc.sulph. 6x
- Silicea 6x

6. Itching, scalp
- Natrum sulph. 6x
- Kali.sulph. 6x
- Calc.sulph. 6x

7. Moist, humid eruptions, on scalp
- Kali.sulph. 6x
- Calc.sulph. 6x
- Silicea 6x

8. Numbness of scalp
- Kali.sulph. 6x
- Kali.phos. 6x
- Calc.sulph. 6x

9. Pustules on scalp
- Natrum sulph. 6x
- Kali.sulph. 6x
- Calc.sulph. 6x

10. Ringworm (Tinea capitis), alopecia areata, bald spots on scalp
- Ferrum phos 6x
- Nat.phos. 6x
- Natrum sulph. 6x

11. Sensitive, to touch, or combing the- scalp
- Kali.phos. 6x
- Natrum sulph. 6x
- Calc.sulph. 6x

12. Sweat, excessive, on scalp
- Natrum sulph. 6x
- Kali.sulph. 6x
- Calc.sulph. 6x

13. Warts, on scalp

Natrum sulph.	6x
Kali.sulph.	6x
Calc.sulph.	6x

SCARLET FEVER (Sore throat, high grade fever and bright red rash all over the body due to streptococcus bacteria)

Kali.sulph.	6x
Calc.sulph.	6x
Silicea	6x

SCHIZOPHRENIA (Psychological disorder with hallucinations, delusions and inability to lead normal life)

Kali.phos.	6x
Calc.sulph.	6x
Silicea	6x

SCIATICA

1. General formula

Calc.phos.	6x
Kali.phos.	6x
Natrum sulph.	6x
Calc.sulph.	6x

2. Left side-sciatica

Natrum sulph.	6x
Kali.sulph.	6x
Calc.sulph.	6x

3. Right side-sciatica

Kali.phos.	6x
Natrum sulph.	6x
Calc.sulph.	6x
Silicea	6x

4. Both sides-sciatica

Ferrum phos	6x
Kali.mur.	6x
Calc.sulph.	6x
Silicea	6x

5. Due to injury, jerk or lifting a weight-sciatica

Kali.phos.	6x
Natrum mur.	6x
Calc.sulph.	6x

6. Due to calcium and vitamin D deficiency-sciatica
   - Kali.sulph. 6x
   - Calc.sulph. 6x
   - Silicea 6x
7. With numbness of leg or foot-sciatica
   - Natrum sulph. 6x
   - Kali.sulph. 6x
   - Calc.sulph. 6x
8. With backache or vertebral disc problem-sciatica
   - Calc.phos. 6x
   - Kali.phos. 6x
   - Ferrum phos 6x
   - Natrum sulph. 6x
9. With wasting of muscles of leg-sciatica
   - Calc.phos. 6x
   - Kali.phos. 6x
   - Calc.sulph. 6x
10. With weakness of legs-sciatica
    - Kali.mur. 6x
    - Calc.sulph. 6x
    - Silicea 6x

SCLERODERMA (hide bound skin-hardening and tightening Of skin and connective tissue)
- Kali.sulph. 6x
- Calc.sulph. 6x
- Silicea 6x

SCLERITIS (inflammation of sclera of eye)
- Calc.phos. 6x
- Natrum sulph. 6x
- Calc.sulph. 6x

SCROFULOUS DISEASES (Tuberculosis, especially in lymph nodes of the neck).
- Calc.phos. 6x
- Natrum sulph. 6x
- Kali sulph. 6x

SCROTUM
1. Eczema-scrotum
   - Kali.mur. 6x
   - Calc.sulph. 6x
   - Silicea 6x
2. Fixed drug eruptions- on scrotum, penis
   - Natrum sulph. 6x
   - Kali.sulph. 6x
   - Calc.sulph. 6x
3. Swelling with collection of fluid in scrotum(Hydrocele)
   - Kali.phos. 6x
   - Kali.sulph. 6x
   - Calc.sulph. 6x

SCURVY (Vitamin C deficiency disease)
- Natrum mur. 6x
- Kali.mur. 6x
- Calc.sulph. 6x

SEA SICKNESS AND TRAVEL SICKNESS
- Ferrum phos 6x
- Natrum sulph. 6x
- Calc.sulph. 6x

SEASONAL FLU - Prevention formula
- Kali.phos. 6x
- Natrum sulph. 6x
- Calc.sulph. 6x

Dose: Once daily for one month before the season starts.

SEASONAL FLU (See Flu, influenza, coryza, cough, fever,
pharyngitis, bronchitis, viral diseases, acute respiratory, distress syndrome, asphyxia, cyanosis, avian influenza, septicemis, bird flu, cyanosis, multiple organ dysfunction syndrome, bronchospam, cough, pneumonia, coma and oxygen-low saturation)

SEBACEOUS CYST

Ferrum phos	6x
Mag.phos.	6x
Natrum sulph.	6x

SEBORRHOEA (Excessive oil production by overactive sebaceous glands in skin; can lead to itching and scales)

Calc.phos.	6x
Kali.phos.	6x
Natrum sulph.	6x

SEBORRHIC DERMATITIS (Itching red patches, greasy scales with white or yellow flakes on skin)

Natrum sulph.	6x
Kali.sulph.	6x
Calc.sulph.	6x

SEMEN (See Sperms also)

1. Bad smell in semen

Kali.phos.	6x
Natrum sulph.	6x
Calc.sulph.	6x

2. Bloody semen

Natrum sulph.	6x
Kali sulph.	6x
Calc.sulph.	6x

3. Less in quantity-semen

Ferrum phos	6x
Natrum sulph.	6x
Calc.sulph.	6x

4. Pus in semen

Kali.sulph.	6x
Calc.sulph.	6x
Silicea	6x

5. Thin semen

Natrum sulph.	6x
Kali.sulph.	6x
Calc.sulph.	6x

(See Sperm disorders also)

SEMINAL VESICULITIS (Inflammation of vesicular glands)
1. Acute vesiculitis

Natrum sulph.	6x
Kali.sulph.	6x
Calc.sulph.	6x

2. Chronic vesiculitis

Calc.phos.	6x
Calc.sulph.	6x
Silicea	6x

SENILE DECAY (aging) (See old age)

SENSATIONS
1. Ants crawling, as if

Kali.phos.	6x
Natrum sulph.	6x
Calc.sulph.	6x

2. Boilig sensation

Natrum sulph.	6x
Kali.sulph.	6x
Calc.sulph.	6x

3. Bubbling sensation

Kali.sulph.	6x
Calc.sulph.	6x
Silicea	6x

4. Burning sensation

Ferrum phos	6x
Natrum sulph.	6x
Calc.sulph.	6x

5. Bursting sensation

Kali.sulph.	6x
Calc.sulph.	6x
Silicea	6x

6. Cold sensation

Calc.sulph.	6x
Calc.flor.	6x
Silicea	6x

7. Constriction sensation
    Kali.mur. 6x
    Calc.flor. 6x
    Silicea 6x

8. Cutting sensation
    Natrum mur. 6x
    Kali.sulph. 6x
    Calc.flor. 6x

9. Enlarged sensation, of a body part
    Kali.sulph. 6x
    Calc.sulph. 6x
    Silicea 6x

10. Hammering sensation
    Kali.phos. 6x
    Mag.phos. 6x
    Calc.sulph. 6x

11. Hot sensation
    Natrum sulph. 6x
    Calc.flor. 6x
    Silicea 6x

12. Needles sensation
    Kali.phos. 6x
    Calc.sulph. 6x
    Silicea 6x

13. Loss of sensation
    Kali.phos. 6x
    Natrum sulph. 6x
    Calc.sulph. 6x

14. Numbness sensation
    Calc.phos. 6x
    Kali.phos. 6x
    Natrum sulph. 6x

15. Pulsating, throbbing sensation
    Natrum mur. 6x
    Natrum sulph. 6x
    Calc.sulph. 6x

16. Trembling sensation, internal
        Calc.sulph. 6x
        Calc.flor. 6x
        Silicea 6x
SEPTICEMIA, SEPTIC SHOCK
        Kali.phos. 6x
        Natrum sulph. 6x
        Kali.sulph. 6x
        Calc.sulph. 6x
SEPTICEMIA, puerperal (during puerperium)
        Natrum sulph. 6x
        Kali.sulph. 6x
        Calc.sulph. 6x
        Silicea 6x
SEPTUM OF NOSE – ulceration (See Nose)

SEPTUM OF HEART, hole in the septum
1. Atrial septal defect (ASD)
        Calc.phos. 6x
        Calc.sulph. 6x
        Calc.flor. 6x
2. Ventricular septal defect (VSD)
        Kali.phos. 6x
        Natrum sulph. 6x
        Calc.flor. 6x
SEIZURES (See Epilesy)
SEVERE ACUTE RESPIRATORY SYNDROME (SARS)
        Natrum sulph. 6x
        Kali.sulph. 6x
        Calc.sulph. 6x
        Silicea 6x
SEXUAL DISORDERS See impotence, Coition also
1. **Emission Disorders**
 a. Emissions (discharge of semen)-In the presence of or thinking about a female
        Kali.phos. 6x
        Natrum sulph. 6x
        Calc.sulph. 6x

b. Emissions- While talking to a female
- Kali.phos. 6x
- Natrum sulph. 6x
- Calc.sulph. 6x

c. Before intercourse
- Kali.mur. 6x
- Kali.sulph. 6x
- Calc.sulph. 6x

d. Emissions-Nocturnal pollutiotions; sexual debility
- Kali.phos. 6x
- Natrum mur. 6x
- Kali.mur. 6x

e. Emissions-With brain-fag, weak legs and backache
- Natrum mur. 6x
- Kali.mur. 6x
- Calc.sulph. 6x

f. Emissions-With emissions, diurnal, straining at stool
- Kali.phos. 6x
- Kali.mur. 6x
- Calc.sulph. 6x

g. With emissions, premature (premature ejaculation)
- Natrum sulph. 6x
- Kali.sulph. 6x
- Calc.sulph. 6x

h. Emissions-With deficient or weak erections
- Kali.sulph. 6x
- Calc.sulph. 6x
- Kali.mur. 6x

i. Emissions-With irritability, despondency, depression
- Calc.sulph. 6x
- Kali.sulph. 6x
- Kali.mur. 6x

2. Penis diseases

a. Atrophy, small in size (children and adults)
- Calc.sulph. 6x
- Kali.phos. 6x
- Natrum sulph. 6x

b. Curved or bent penis (See Peyronie's disease also)
  Kali.phos. 6x
  Natrum sulph. 6x
  Calc.sulph. 6x
3. **Erection problems**
a. Erectile dysfunction (ED)
  Kali.phos. 6x
  Natrum mur. 6x
  Kali.sulph. 6x
  Calc.sulph. 6x
b. Erection goes away during coition
  Kali.phos. 6x
  Natrum sulph. 6x
  Calc.sulph. 6x
  Silicea 6x
c. No erection at all
  Natrum sulph. 6x
  Calc.sulph. 6x
  Silicea 6x
d. Premature ejaculation (PE)
  Natrum sulph. 6x
  Kali.sulph. 6x
  Calc.sulph. 6x
e. Weak erections
  Kali.phos. 6x
  Natrum sulph. 6x
  Kali.sulph. 6x
  Calc.sulph. 6x
4. **Sexual desire - Males**
a. Increased or excessive sex desire (Satyriasis)
  Natrum sulph. 6x
  Kali.sulph. 6x
  Calc.sulph. 6x
b. Gone or Lost-sexual desire
  Kali.sulph. 6x
  Calc.sulph. 6x
  Silicea 30x

5. **Sexual desire - Females**
a. Increased or excessive (Nymhomania)
   - Kali.phos. 6x
   - Natrum sulph. 6x
   - Calc.sulph. 6x
b. Loss of sexual desire (Frigidity)
   - Kali.phos. 6x
   - Natrum mur. 6x
   - Kali.mur. 30x

SEXUALLY TRANSMITTED DISEASES (STDs)

1. AIDS (acquired immunodeficiency syndrome)
   - Kali.mur. 6x
   - Kali.sulph. 6x
   - Calc.sulph. 6x
2. Bacterial vaginosis
   - Kali.sulph. 6x
   - Calc.sulph. 6x
   - Calc.flor. 6x
   - Silicea 6x
3. Chlamydia infection
   - Natrum sulph. 6x
   - Kali.mur. 6x
   - Kali sulph. 6x
4. Genital herpes
   - Natrum sulph. 6x
   - Kali.sulph. 6x
   - Calc.sulph. 6x
5. Gonorrhea (see gonorrhea also)
   - Kali.sulph. 6x
   - Calc.sulph. 6x
   - Silicea 6x
6. Human paipilloma virus (HPV) infection
   - Kali.phos. 6x
   - Natrum sulph. 6x
   - Calc.sulph. 6x

7. Pelvic inflammatory disease (see pelvic diseases)
   - Kali.phos. 6x
   - Kali.sulph. 6x
   - Calc.sulph. 6x
   - Silicea 6x
8. Syphilis
   - Kali.sulph. 6x
   - Calc.sulph. 6x
   - Silicea 6x
9. Trichomonas infection
   - Natrum mur. 6x
   - Kali.mur. 6x
   - Calc.sulph. 6x

SHIGELLOSIS (Bacillary dysentery)
- Natrum sulph. 6x
- Kali.sulph. 6x
- Calc.sulph. 6x

SHINGLES (Herpes zoster)
- Natrum sulph. 6x
- Kali.mur. 6x
- Kali sulph. 6x

SHOCK DUE TO INJURY OR ACCIDENT
- Natrum sulph. 6x
- Kali.mur. 6x
- Calc.sulph. 6x

SHOULDER
1. Dislocation of shoulder joint
   - Natrum mur. 6x
   - Kali.mur. 6x
   - Calc.sulph. 6x
2. Frozen shoulder
   - Kali.phos. 6x
   - Natrum sulph. 6x
   - Kali sulph. 6x
3. Injury or sprain of shoulder capsule or tendons
   - Natrum sulph. 6x
   - Kali.sulph. 6x
   - Calc.sulph. 6x

SINUSITIS

1. General formula
   - Calc.phos. 6x
   - Ferrum phos 6x
   - Calc.sulph. 6x
2. Ethmoidal sinusitis
   - Natrum sulph. 6x
   - Kali.sulph. 6x
   - Calc.sulph. 6x
3. Frontal sinuses, inflammation (frontal sinusitis)
   - Natrum sulph. 6x
   - Kali.sulph. 6x
   - Calc.sulph. 6x
4. Antrum, pain and swelling (maxillary sinusitis)
   - Calc.phos. 6x
   - Kali.phos. 6x
   - Natrum sulph. 6x
5. Fungal sinusitis
   - Natrum mur. 6x
   - Kali.mur. 6x
   - Calc.sulph. 6x
6. Sphenoid sinusitis
   - Kali.phos. 6x
   - Natrum mur. 6x
   - Calc.sulph. 6x

SJOGREN'S SYNDROME (Dryness of eyes and mouth)
- Calc.phos. 6x
- Natrum mur. 6x
- Kali.mur. 6x

SKIN DISEASES (See Acne, Baker's itch, Barber's itch, Comedo, Dermatitis, Eczema, Ecchymoses, Frackles, Furuncles, Fungal infection, Leucoderma, Petechiae, Pityriasis, Pruritus, Psoriasis, Ringworm, Scalp, Swimmer's itch, Warts).

SLEEP APNOEA (Breathing stops on going to sleep)

	Kali.phos.	3x
	Kali.sulph.	3x
	Natrum sulph.	3x

SLEEPLESSNESS (Insomnia)

1. General formula

Natrum sulph.	6x
Calc.sulph.	6x
Silicea	6x

2. Children

Ferrum phos	6x
Natrum sulph.	6x
Calc.sulph.	6x

3. Old age

Kali.sulph.	6x
Calc.sulph.	6x
Silicea	6x

SLEEPLESSNESS - DUE TO

1. Alcohol, drugs abuse

Calc.sulph.	6x
Natrum sulph.	6x
Kali.phos.	6x

2. Arterial pulsations

Kali.sulph.	6x
Calc.sulph.	6x
Calc.flor.	6x

3. Body pain and aches

Kali.sulph.	6x
Calc.sulph.	6x
Silicea	6x

4. Chronic diseases (diabetes, hypertension, arthritis)

Natrum sulph.	6x
Kali.sulph.	6x
Calc.sulph.	6x

5. Difficulty in falling to sleep
   - Kali.phos. 6x
   - Kali.sulph. 6x
   - Calc.sulph. 6x
6. Difficulty in falling to sleep, if wakes up during sleep
   - Natrum mur. 6x
   - Kali.mur. 6x
   - Calc.sulph. 6x
7. Disppointment or depression
   - Kali.phos. 6x
   - Natrum sulph. 6x
   - Calc.sulph. 6x
8. Financial loss
   - Natrum sulph. 6x
   - Kali.sulph. 6x
   - Silicea 6x
9. Financial problems
   - Kali.phos. 6x
   - Kali.mur. 6x
   - Silicea 6x
10. Hypertension
    - Kali.phos. 6x
    - Natrum sulph. 6x
    - Calc.sulph. 6x
11. Mental strain
    - Natrum sulph. 6x
    - Calc.sulph. 6x
    - Silicea 6x
12. Persistent thoughts, in mind
    - Kali.phos. 6x
    - Calc.sulph. 6x
    - Natrum sulph. 6x
13. Post-traumatic stress disorder (PTSD)
    - Natrum sulph. 6x
    - Kali.sulph. 6x
    - Calc.sulph. 6x

14. Psychological trauma or shock
    - Kali.phos. 6x
    - Natrum sulph. 6x
    - Calc.sulph. 6x

15. Shock in abuse victims, siege and war victims
    - Kali.phos. 6x
    - Natrum sulph. 6x
    - Kali.sulph. 6x
    - Calc.sulph. 6x

16. Shock, in rape or abuse victims
    - Natrum sulph. 6x
    - Kali.sulph. 6x
    - Calc.sulph. 6x
    - Silicea 6x

17. Weakness
    - Calc.phos. 6x
    - Kali.phos. 6x
    - Silicea 6x

SLEEP - EXCESSIVE
- Natrum mur. 6x
- Kali.mur. 6x
- Calc.sulph. 6x

SLEEP WALKING (Somnambulism)
- Natrum sulph. 6x
- Kali.sulph. 6x
- Calc.sulph. 6x

SMALLPOX (Variola)
- Natrum sulph. 6x
- Kali.sulph. 6x
- Calc.sulph. 6x

SMELL DISORDERS

1. Sense of smell - diminished
   - Calc.phos. 6x
   - Kali.phos. 6x
   - Natrum mur. 6x

2. Hypersensitive to flowers, food, etc
  Kali.phos. 6x
  Natrum mur. 6x
  Kali.mur. 6x
3. Lost (anosmia) or perverted
  Kali.phos. 6x
  Natrum sulph. 6x
  Calc.sulph. 6x
4. Imaginary smells (olfactory hallucinations)
  Calc.phos. 6x
  Kali.phos. 6x
  Calc.sulph. 6x

SMOKING HABIT-To Remove
  Kali.phos. 6x
  Natrum sulph. 6x
  Calc.sulph. 6x

SNEEZING - all types (See Allergy, Hay fever, Nose, Rhinitis also)
  Kali.phos. 6x
  Natrum sulph. 6x
  Calc.sulph. 6x

SOMATOFORM DISORDERS (Somatic system disorders-SSD)
1. Anxiety disorders
  Kali.phos. 6x
  Natrum sulph. 6x
  Kali sulph. 6x
2. Body dysmorphic disorder
  Kali.phos. 6x
  Natrum sulph. 6x
  Calc.sulph. 6x
3. Conversion disorder (Functional neurological symptom disorder)-without any medical cause.
 a. Abnormal movements (tremors, seizures, walking disorders)
  Natrum sulph. 6x
  Kali.sulph. 6x
  Calc.sulph. 6x

b. Blindness

    Natrum sulph. 6x
    Kali.sulph. 6x
    Calc.sulph. 6x

c. Hearing loss

    Kali.phos. 6x
    Natrum sulph. 6x
    Calc.sulph. 6x

d. Sensory loss (loss of sensation)

    Natrum sulph. 6x
    Calc.sulph. 6x
    Silicea 6x

e. Weakness

    Natrum sulph. 6x
    Kali.sulph. 6x
    Calc.sulph. 6x

4. Distress

    Kali.phos. 6x
    Natrum sulph. 6x
    Calc.sulph. 6x

5. False belief of pregnancy (Pseudocyesis) and feeling all signs of pregnancy, like movement of fetus, etc.

    Calc.sulph. 6x
    Kali.sulph. 6x
    Natrum sulph. 6x

6. Gastrointestinal problems

    Natrum sulph. 6x
    Calc.sulph. 6x
    Silicea 6x

7. Hypochondriasis

    Kali.phos. 6x
    Natrum sulph. 6x
    Calc.sulph. 6x

8. Illness anxiety disorder (Hypochondriasis)-Patient thinks that minor symptoms are signs of very serious disease. i.e., his headache is due to brain tumor.
  Kali.phos. 6x
  Natrum sulph. 6x
  Calc.sulph. 6x

9. Neurological disorders
  Natrum sulph. 6x
  Kali.sulph. 6x
  Calc.sulph. 6x

10. Pain
  Kali.phos. 6x
  Natrum sulph. 6x
  Calc.sulph. 6x

11. Sexual problems
  Kali.phos. 6x
  Natrum mur. 6x
  Calc.sulph. 6x

SORE THROAT
  Kali.phos. 6x
  Kali.mur. 6x
  Calc.sulph. 6x

SPASMS, CONVULSIONS
  Kali.phos. 6x
  Natrum sulph. 6x
  Calc.sulph. 6x

SPERMATIC CORDS - pain, inflammation (Funiculitis)
  Kali.phos. 6x
  Kali.sulph. 6x
  Calc.sulph. 6x

SPERM DISORDERS
1. Absence of sperms (Azoospermia)
  Kali.phos. 6x
  Kali.sulph. 6x
  Calc.sulph. 6x
  Natrum sulph. 6x

2. Bloody semen
- Natrum sulph. 6x
- Kali sulph. 6x
- Calc.sulph. 6x

3. Poor motility of sperms
- Kali.phos. 6x
- Kali.sulph. 6x
- Calc.sulph. 6x
- Silicea 6x

4. Less number of sperms (Oligospermia)
- Kali.phos. 6x
- Natrum sulph. 6x
- Calc.sulph. 6x

5. Poor quality of sperms (asthenospermia-weak sperms)
- Kali.phos. 6x
- Natrum sulph. 6x
- Kali.sulph. 6x
- Calc.sulph. 6x

6. Stenosis (narrowing) of spermatic cord or blockage
- Natrum sulph. 6x
- Kali.sulph. 6x
- Calc.sulph. 6x

7. Teratospermia (sperms of abnormal shapes)
- Kali.phos. 6x
- Natrum mur. 6x
- Calc.sulph. 6x

8. Thin semen
- Natrum sulph. 6x
- Kali.sulph. 6x
- Calc.sulph. 6x

SPERMATORRHOEA (Involuntary loss of semen)

1. Spermatorrhoea and after-effects
   - a. Kali.phos. 6x
     - Natrum sulph. 6x
     - Kali.sulph. 6x
     - Calc.sulph. 6x
   - b. Kali.phos. 6x
     - Calc.phos. 6x

2. With debility, weak legs, backache
  Ferrum phos. 6x
  Kali.phos. 6x
  Mag.phos. 6x
  Kali.sulph. 6x
  Calc.sulph. 6x
3. With emissions, premature
  Kali.phos. 6x
  Natrum sulph. 6x
  Kali.sulph. 6x
  Calc.sulph. 6x
4. With weak erections
  Kali.phos. 6x
  Natrum sulph. 6x
  Calc.sulph. 6x
  Silicea 6x

SPINAL CORD (See Myelitis)
SPINE DISEASES (See Back, Backache, Sciatica, Disc)
1. Bulging of vertebral disc
  Calc.sulph. 6x
  Natrum sulph. 6x
  Calc.flor. 6x
2. Degenerative disc disorders
  Kali.phos. 6x
  Natrum sulph. 6x
  Calc.sulph. 6x
3. Hyperaesthesia (excessive sensitivity)
  Kali.phos. 6x
  Kali.sulph. 6x
  Calc.sulph. 6x
4. Hyperaesthesia (excessive sensitivity), from using arms in sewing, typewriting, etc.
  Kali.phos. 6x
  Kali.mur. 6x
  Kali.sulph. 6x
  Calc.sulph. 6x

5. Hyperaesthesia, sits sideways to prevent pressure on spine

Kali.phos.	6x
Natrum sulph.	6x
Kali.sulph.	6x
Calc.sulph.	6x

6. Inflammation of spinal cord (Acute Myelitis)

Kali.phos.	6x
Kali.sulph.	6x
Calc.sulph.	6x

7. Inflammation of spinal cord (Chronic Myelitis)

Natrum sulph.	6x
Kali.sulph.	6x
Calc.sulph.	6x

8. Injury of spinal cord (spinal concussion)

Kali.phos.	6x
Natrum sulph.	6x
Calc.sulph.	6x

9. Stenosis (narrowing) of spinal canal

Kali.sulph.	6x
Calc.sulph.	6x
Silicea	6x

SPLEEN - DISEASES

1. Atrophy, contracted, induration

Natrum sulph.	6x
Kali.sulph.	6x
Calc.sulph.	6x

2. Clots in the vein of spleen

Natrum sulph.	6x
Kali.sulph.	6x
Calc.sulph.	6x

3. Enlargement of spleen (Splenomegaly)

Ferrum phos	6x
Natrum sulph.	6x
Calc.sulph.	6x

4. Inflammation (Splenitis)

Natrum sulph.	6x
Kali.sulph.	6x
Calc.sulph.	6x

5. Pain in spleen

Kali.sulph.	6x
Calc.sulph.	6x
Silicea	6x

SPRAIN, STRAIN

1. General formula (all types of sprains)

Kali.phos.	6x
Natrum sulph.	6x
Calc.sulph.	6x

2. Back-sprain

Kali.phos.	6x
Natrum sulph.	6x
Kali.sulph.	6x
Calc.sulph.	6x

3. Joints-sprain

Natrum sulph.	6x
Calc.sulph.	6x
Silicea	6x

4. Muscles-sprain

Calc.phos.	6x
Kali.phos.	6x
Calc.sulph.	6x

5. Tendons-sprain

Calc.sulph.	6x
Kali.sulph.	6x
Silicea	6x

STAGE FRIGHT

Kali.phos.	6x
Kali.sulph.	6x
Calc.sulph.	6x

STERILITY- FEMALES & MALES

Kali.phos.	6x
Natrum sulph.	6x
Kali.sulph.	6x
Calc.sulph.	6x

STEVEN JOHNSON SYNDROME

Kali.phos.	6x
Kali.sulph.	6x
Calc.sulph.	6x

Dose: In serious cases give 2 hourly, for 2 days; then give 4 times daily.

STOMACH, DISEASES

1. Acidity, burning in stomach

Natrum sulph.	6x
Kali.sulph.	6x
Calc.sulph.	6x

2. Dilatation of stomach (gastroptosis)

Natrum sulph.	6x
Kali.sulph.	6x
Calc.sulph.	6x
Silicea	6x

3. Cardiac orifice of stomach-contraction

Natrum sulph.	6x
Kali.mur.	6x
Calc.sulph.	6x

4. Haemorrhage from stomach (Haemetemesis)

Natrum sulph.	6x
Kali.sulph.	6x
Calc.sulph.	6x

5. Pain (See Gastric Pain)

STOMATITIS (inflammation and soreness of mouth)

Natrum sulph.	6x
Kali.mur.	6x
Calc.sulph.	6x

STRABISMUS (Squint eyes)
1. General formula

Kali.phos.	6x
Natrum sulph.	6x
Calc.sulph.	6x

2. Convergent squint (eye balls turned inwards)

Calc.sulph.	6x
Natrum sulph.	6x
Kali.phos.	6x

3. Divergent squint (eye balls turned outwards)

Natrum sulph.	6x
Calc.sulph.	6x
Calc.flor.	6x

4. Due to intestinal worms-squint occurs

Natrum sulph.	6x
Kali.sulph.	6x
Calc.sulph.	6x

STRANGURY (Painful, frequent urination, in small quantities)

Natrum sulph.	6x
Kali.sulph.	6x
Calc.sulph.	6x

STYE (pus filled reddish boil on edge of eyelid due to blockage of a gland or a follicle)

Natrum sulph.	6x
Kali.sulph.	6x
Calc.sulph.	6x

SUN STROKE

Ferrum phos	6x
Natrum mur.	6x
Calc.sulph.	6x

SUPPRESSED SEXUAL DESIRE, ill-effects of

Kali.phos. 6x
Kali.sulph. 6x
Calc.sulph. 6x

SUPPURATION (Easy tendency to pus formation)

Calc.sulph. 6x
Kali.sulph. 6x
Natrum sulph. 6x

(See Abscess also)

SURGERY

Before surgey give (2 doses at 3 hours interval)

Kali.sulph. 6x
Calc.sulph. 6x
Silicea 6x

After surgery give (3-4 times a day for one week)

Kali.phos. 6x
Natrum sulph. 6x
Calc.sulph. 6x

SURGICAL SHOCK

Kali.phos. 6x
Natrum sulph. 6x
Kali.sulph. 6x
Calc.sulph. 6x

Repeat after every 5 minute till improvement occurs.

SWEAT DISORDERS

1. Absence of sweating (anidrosis)

Kali.phos. 6x
Kali.mur. 6x
Calc.sulph. 6x

2. Cold, clammy sweat

Kali.phos. 6x
Natrum sulph. 6x
Calc.sulph. 6x

3. Hands-palms, sweating
 - Kali.phos. 6x
 - Natrum sulph. 6x
 - Calc.sulph. 6x

4. Head, excessive sweating
 - Silicea 6x
 - Kali.sulph. 6x
 - Calc.sulph. 6x

5. Head, occipital region (back of head), excessive
 - Calc.sulph. 6x
 - Kali.sulph. 6x
 - Natrum sulph. 6x

6. Increased, all over body-sweating
   a.
 - Kali.sulph. 6x
 - Natrum sulph. 6x
 - Calc.sulph. 6x
   b.
 - Calc.phos. 6x
 - Natrum. mur. 6x
 - Silicea 6x

7. Increased, in axillae-sweating
 - Kali.phos. 6x
 - Natrum sulph. 6x
 - Calc.sulph. 6x

8. On face, forehead-excess sweating
 - Kali.phos. 6x
 - Natrum sulph. 6x
 - Calc.sulph. 6x

9. On feet, sweating, with offensive smell
 - Kali.phos. 6x
 - Natrum sulph. 6x
 - Silicea 6x

10. On genital organs-excess sweating
 - Kali.phos. 6x
 - Natrum sulph. 6x
 - Calc.sulph. 6x

SWEAT, ODOR
1. Foetid, offensive, bad smelling sweat

    Kali.phos.   6x
    Natrum sulph.   6x
    Calc.sulph.   6x

2. Sour, acrid, acidic sweat, irritating the skin

    Natrum sulph.   6x
    Kali.sulph.   6x
    Calc.sulph.   6x

SWEATING, relieves the symptoms

    Kali.phos.   6x
    Natrum sulph.   6x
    Calc.sulph.   6x

SWIMMER'S ITCH (skin rash due to allergic reaction of skin to micro-parasites, released by infected snails in water)

    Kali.phos.   6x
    Natrum sulph.   6x
    Calc.sulph.   6x

SWINE FLU, Swine flu in humans (H3 N2 virus)

    Kali.sulph.   6x
    Calc.sulph.   6x
    Calc.flor.   6x
    Silicea   6x

SYCOSIS (See Barber's itch)

SYNCOPE-FAINTING: CAUSES
1. Dehydration

    Natrum mur.   6x
    Kali.mur.   6x
    Calc.sulph.   6x

2. Heat, excessive or heat stroke

    Natrum sulph.   6x
    Calc.sulph.   6x
    Silicea   6x

3. Hysterical tendency of syncope

	Kali.phos.	6x
	Natrum sulph.	6x
	Calc.sulph.	6x

4. Irregular heart beat, cardiac arrhythmia-syncope

	Natrum sulph.	6x
	Kali.sulph.	6x
	Silicea	6x

5. Vaso-vagal syncope (neuro-cardiogenic syncope)

	Kali.phos.	6x
	Kali.sulph.	6x
	Silicea	6x

SYNOVITIS (inflammation of the synoial membrane lining the inner cavity of joints)

1. Acute synovitis

	Natrum sulph.	6x
	Kali.sulph.	6x
	Calc.sulph.	6x

2. Chronic synovitis

	Natrum sulph.	6x
	Kali.sulph.	6x
	Silicea	6x

SYPHILIS
    General formula

	Kali.sulph.	6x
	Calc.sulph.	6x
	Silicea	6x

SYPHILIS – Long term Comlpications

1. Adenopathy, lymph node swelling-due to syphilis

	Kali.sulph.	6x
	Calc.sulph.	6x
	Silicea	6x

2. Alopecia (hair falling)-due to syphilis

	Natrum sulph.	6x
	Kali.sulph.	6x
	Calc.sulph.	6x

3. Arthritis-due to syphilis
- Ferrum phos 6x
- Natrum sulph. 6x
- Calc.sulph. 6x

4. Blood vessles, degeneration-due to syphilis
- Kali.phos. 6x
- Natrum sulph. 6x
- Calc.sulph. 6x

5. Bone and cartilage damage-due to syphilis
- Natrum sulph. 6x
- Kali.sulph. 6x
- Silicea 6x

6. Brain degeneration-due to syphilis
- Kali.sulph. 6x
- Calc.sulph. 6x
- Silicea 6x

7. Condylomata lata (sign of secondary syphilis)
- Natrum sulph. 6x
- Calc.sulph. 6x
- Kali sulph. 6x

8. Eyes diseases-due to syphilis
- Calc.phos. 6x
- Natrum sulph. 6x
- Calc.sulph. 6x

9. Gummata, nodes-due to syphilis
- Kali.sulph. 6x
- Calc.sulph. 6x
- Silicea 6x

10. Headache-due to syphilis
- Natrum sulph. 6x
- Kali.sulph. 6x
- Silicea 6x

11. Heart diseases-due to syphilis
- Kali.phos. 6x
- Natrum sulph. 6x
- Calc.sulph. 6x

12. Liver damage-due to syphilis
    - Kali.sulph. 6x
    - Calc.sulph. 6x
    - Silicea 6x
13. Mucous patches or ulcers-due to syphilis
    - Kali.phos. 6x
    - Kali.mur. 6x
    - Calc.sulph. 6x
14. Neurological disorders-due to syphilis
    - Natrum sulph. 6x
    - Kali.sulph. 6x
    - Calc.sulph. 6x
15. Nocturnal pain in bones and joints-due to syphilis
    - Kali.sulph. 6x
    - Calc.sulph. 6x
    - Silicea 6x

(See Tabes dorsalis as well)

SYSTEMIC LUPUS ERYTHEMATOSUS (SLE)
- Natrum sulph. 6x
- Kali.sulph. 6x
- Calc.sulph. 6x

T

TABES DORSALIS (neurosyphilis, signs of tertiary syphilis)

1. General formula
 - Kali.sulph. 6x
 - Calc.sulph. 6x
 - Silicea 6x

2. Abnormal gait or unable to walk (Locomotor ataxia)
 - Kali.phos. 6x
 - Natrum sulph. 6x
 - Calc.sulph. 6x

3. Depression - due to tertiary syphilis
 - Kali.phos. 6x
 - Natrum sulph. 6x
 - Calc.sulph. 6x

4. Headache - due to tertiary syphilis
 - Kali.phos. 6x
 - Mag.phos. 6x
 - Calc.sulph. 6x

5. Irritability - due to tertiary syphilis
 - Kali.mur. 6x
 - Kali.sulph. 6x
 - Calc.sulph. 6x

6. Loss of urine control (urinary incontinence)
 - Kali.phos. 6x
 - Kali.sulph. 6x
 - Calc.sulph. 6x

7. Nerves damage - due to tertiary syphilis
 - Kali.phos. 6x
 - Calc.sulph. 6x
 - Natrum sulph. 6x

8. Numbness in legs, feet or toes - due to tertiary syphilis
 - Kali.phos. 6x
 - Natrum mur. 6x
 - Calc.sulph. 6x

9. Problems in thinking and concentration-in tertiary syphilis

Kali.phos.	6x
Kali.sulph.	6x
Calc.sulph.	6x

10. Seizures, fits - due to tertiary syphilis

Kali.phos.	6x
Natrum sulph.	6x
Calc.sulph.	6x

11. Spinal cord damage - due to tertiary syphilis

Kali.phos.	6x
Natrum sulph.	6x
Calc.sulph.	6x

12. Stiff neck - due to tertiary syphilis

Kali.phos.	6x
Natrum mur.	6x
Calc.sulph.	6x

13. Tremors-hands and body - due to tertiary syphilis

Kali.phos.	6x
Natrum mur.	6x
Kali.sulph.	6x

14. Weakness - due to tertiary syphilis

Kali.sulph.	6x
Calc.sulph.	6x
Silicea	6x

TACHYCARDIA (rapid pulse) (See Pulse)

TAENIA (tapeworm) (See Worms)

TARSAL TUNNEL SYNDROME (pain one inner side of ankle and foot due to compression of posterior tibial nerve)

Natrum mur.	6x
Kali.sulph.	6x
Calc.sulph.	6x

TASTE, DISORDERS

1. Bad taste
   - Kali.phos. 6x
   - Natrum sulph. 6x
   - Calc.sulph. 6x

2. Loss of taste
   - Kali.phos. 6x
   - Kali.mur. 6x
   - Calc.sulph. 6x

3. Perverted, altered taste
   - Kali.phos. 6x
   - Natrum sulph. 6x
   - Calc.sulph. 6x

4. Bitter, bilious taste
   - Natrum sulph. 6x
   - Kali.sulph. 6x
   - Calc.sulph. 6x

5. Disgusting, foul taste
   - Kali.phos. 6x
   - Natrum sulph. 6x
   - Silicea 6x

6. Greasy, fatty taste
   - Kali.phos. 6x
   - Natrum sulph. 6x
   - Calc.sulph. 6x

7. Metallic taste
   - Natrum sulph. 6x
   - Kali.sulph. 6x
   - Calc.sulph. 6x

8. Sour taste
   - Kali.phos. 6x
   - Kali.mur. 6x
   - Calc.sulph. 6x

TEMPORO – MANDIBULAR JOINT DISEASE

1. Arthritis of TMJ
   - Kali.phos. 6x
   - Kali.sulph. 6x
   - Calc.sulph. 6x
2. Cracking sound-temporo-mandiular joint
   - Calc.phos. 6x
   - Kali.phos. 6x
   - Calc.sulph. 6x
3. Dislocated easily - TM joint
   - Kali.phos. 6x
   - Natrum sulph. 6x
   - Calc.sulph. 6x
4. Pain in TM joint
   - Kali.phos. 6x
   - Kali.sulph. 6x
   - Calc.sulph. 6x

TENESMUS IN URINARY BLADDER (See Strangury also)
- Natrum sulph. 6x
- Kali.sulph. 6x
- Calc.sulph. 6x

Tenesmus, with painful urging of urination
- Kali.sulph. 6x
- Natrum sulph. 6x
- Calc.sulph. 6x

TENESMUS IN RECTUM
- Ferrum phos 6x
- Kali.sulph. 6x
- Calc.sulph. 6x

TENNIS ELBOW (Pain in outer side of elbow due to lateral epicondylitis)
- Mag.phos. 6x
- Calc.sulph. 6x
- Natrum mur. 6x

TENO-SYNOVITIS (inflammation of internal lining of the sheath which surrounds the tendon)

    Kali.phos. 6x
    Natrum sulph. 6x
    Calc.sulph. 6x

TEETH - DISEASES

1. Alveolar abscess (abscess in bony socket of tooth)
    Kali.sulph. 6x
    Calc.sulph. 6x
    Silicea 6x
2. Caries (decay) of teeth
    Natrum sulph. 6x
    Kali.sulph. 6x
    Calc.sulph. 6x
3. Caries (decay) at crown of tooth
    Kali.phos. 6x
    Natrum sulph. 6x
    Calc.sulph. 6x
4. Craies (decay) at root of tooth
    Kali.sulph. 6x
    Calc.sulph. 6x
    Silicea 6x

5. Teeth - Feel loose in sockets
    Kali.phos. 6x
    Natrum sulph. 6x
    Calc.sulph. 6x
6. Teeth - Sensitive to cold, chewing, touch
    Silicea 6x
    Kali.sulph. 6x
    Calc.sulph. 6x
7. Teeth - Sensitive to hot items
    Calc.sulph. 6x
    Kali sulph. 6x
    Silicea 6x

8. Teeth - grinding

Kali.phos.	6x
Natrum mur.	6x
Calc.sulph.	6x

9. Teeth - grinding and clenching jaws

Kali.phos.	6x
Calc.sulph.	6x
Silicea	6x

10. Teeth, sordes, deposits and black spots

Kali.sulph.	6x
Calc.sulph.	6x
Silicea	6x

TEETHING PROBLEMS - CHILDREN

1. Delayed teething (dentition)

Kali.phos.	6x
Natrum sulph.	6x
Calc.sulph.	6x

2. Teething, delayed with diarrhoea

Natrum sulph.	6x
Kali.sulph.	6x
Calc.sulph.	6x

3. Teething with resltlessness, irritability, fever

Ferrum phos	6x
Natrum sulph.	6x
Calc.sulph.	6x

TENDINITIS

Kali.sulph.	6x
Calc.sulph.	6x
Calc.flor.	6x

TESTES

1. Abscess

Kali.phos.	6x
Natrum sulph.	6x
Calc.sulph.	6x

2. Atrophy of testes

Kali.phos.	6x
Calc.sulph.	6x
Calc.flor.	6x

3. Hypertrophy of testes
   - Kali.phos. 6x
   - Natrum sulph. 6x
   - Calc.sulph. 6x
4. Epididymitis
   - Kali.phos. 6x
   - Natrum sulph. 6x
   - Calc.sulph. 6x
   - Silicea 6x
5. Orchitis (inflammation the testicles)
   - Natrum sulph. 6x
   - Kali.sulph. 6x
   - Calc.sulph. 6x
6. Pain in testes
   - Kali.sulph. 6x
   - Calc.sulph. 6x
   - Silicea 6x
7. Tumor of testes
   - Natrum sulph. 6x
   - Kali.sulph. 6x
   - Calc.sulph. 6x
   - Silicea 6x
8. Undescended testes
   - Kali.phos. 6x
   - Natrum sulph. 6x
   - Calc.sulph. 6x
   - Silicea 6x

TETANUS (Curative and preventive formulas)
- Calc.phos. 6x
- Kali.sulph. 6x
- Calc.sulph. 6x

Prevention: Once in a week for 3 months.
Treatment: One dose after every half hour, for 6 hours;then give 4 times daily for one week.

THALASSEMIA

Ferrum phos	6x
Natrum sulph.	6x
Calc.sulph.	6x

THIGH - PAIN

Calc.phos.	6x
Natrum mur.	6x
Kali sulph.	6x

THIRST

1. Excessive thirst

Natrum sulph.	6x
Kali.sulph.	6x
Calc.sulph.	6x

2. Thirstlessness

Kali.phos.	6x
Kali.mur.	6x
Calc.sulph.	6x

THROMBO – EMBOLISM, IN ARTERIES

Natrum sulph.	6x
Kali sulph.	6x
Calc.sulph.	6x

THROMBOPHLEBITIS

Kali.phos.	6x
Natrum sulph.	6x
Calc.sulph.	6x

THRMBOSIS - CORONARY and Angina pectoris

Natrum sulph.	6x
Kali.sulph.	6x
Calc.sulph.	6x

THYROID GLAND (See Goitre)

TINEA BARBAE (See Barber's itch)

TINEA CAPITIS (Fungus on scalp)

Ferrum phos	6x
Natrum sulph.	6x
Calc.sulph.	6x

TINEA VERSICOLOR (Pityriasis versicolor)

Natrum mur.	6x
Kali.sulph.	6x
Calc.sulph.	6x

TINNITUS AURIUM (Noise in ears) - TYPES

1. General formula

Kali.phos.	6x
Natrum sulph.	6x
Calc.sulph.	6x

2. Hissing sound

Natrum sulph.	6x
Kali.sulph.	6x
Calc.sulph.	6x

3. Humming sound

Natrum sulph.	6x
Calc.sulph.	6x
Silicea	6x

4. Re - echoing of voice or sounds

Natrum sulph.	6x
Kali.mur.	6x
Calc.flor.	6x

5. Ringing of bells

Kali.phos.	6x
Kali.mur.	6x
Calc.sulph.	6x

6. Whizzing sound

Calc.phos.	6x
Ferrum phos	6x
Kali.sulph.	6x
Calc.sulph.	6x

TINNITUS AURIUM - CAUSES

1. Arteriosclerosis of blood vessels of ear

Kali.phos.	6x
Natrum sulph.	6x
Calc.sulph.	6x

2. Diabetic patients
   - Calc.phos. 6x
   - Kali.phos. 6x
   - Natrum mur. 6x
3. Ear infections
   - Natrum sulph. 6x
   - Kali.sulph. 6x
   - Calc.sulph. 6x
4. Grief
   - Kali.phos. 6x
   - Natrum mur. 6x
   - Kali.mur. 6x
5. Head injury - effects of
   - Kali.phos. 6x
   - Natrum sulph. 6x
   - Calc.sulph. 6x
6. Hypertension cases
   - Kali.phos. 6x
   - Natrum sulph. 6x
   - Calc.sulph. 6x
7. Old age - ear noises, due to
   - Kali.phos. 6x
   - Natrum sulph. 6x
   - Calc.sulph. 6x

TOBACCO - ABUSE

1. Ill-effects of tobacco abuse
   - Calc.phos. 6x
   - Kali.phos. 6x
   - Natrum sulph. 6x
2. To quit the habit of toabacco abuse
   - Ferrum phos 6x
   - Natrum sulph. 6x
   - Calc.sulph. 6x

TONGUE - Coating, Color

1. Balck coating
   - Kali.phos. 6x
   - Natrum sulph. 6x
   - Calc.sulph. 6x
2. Bluish coating
   - Natrum sulph. 6x
   - Calc.sulph. 6x
   - Silicea 6x
3. Brownish coating
   - Kali.phos. 6x
   - Kali.mur. 6x
   - Calc.sulph. 6x
4. Dirty coating
   - Kali.sulph. 6x
   - Calc.sulph. 6x
   - Silicea 6x
5. Greenish coating
   - Kali.sulph. 6x
   - Calc.sulph. 6x
   - Natrum sulph. 6x
6. Mapped tongue
   - Kali.mur. 6x
   - Kali.sulph. 6x
   - Calc.sulph. 6x
7. Red, raw tongue
   - Natrum sulph. 6x
   - Kali.sulph. 6x
   - Calc.sulph. 6x
8. White, furred tongue
   - Kali.phos. 6x
   - Natrum sulph. 6x
   - Calc.sulph. 6x
9. Yellow, dirty, thick coating, on tongue
   - Calc.phos. 6x
   - Ferrum phos 6x
   - Natrum sulph. 6x

TONGUE, ERUPTIONS, GROWTHS

1. Cancer of tongue

Ferrum phos	6x
Natrum mur.	6x
Kali.mur.	6x
Calc.sulph.	6x

2. Cracks, excoriation of tongue

Natrum sulph.	6x
Kali.sulph.	6x
Calc.sulph.	6x

3. Growths, nodules on tongue

Calc.flor.	6x
Kali.sulph.	6x
Calc.sulph.	6x

4. Ulcers on tongue

Kali.sulph.	6x
Calc.sulph.	6x
Silicea	6x

TONGUE - DISORDERS

1. Biting the tongue, while chewing or talking

Kali.phos.	6x
Natrum sulph.	6x
Calc.sulph.	6x

2. Dryness of tongue

Natrum sulph.	6x
Kali.sulph.	6x
Calc.sulph.	6x

3. Inflammation of tongue (Glossitis)

Natrum sulph.	6x
Kali.sulph.	6x
Calc.sulph.	6x

4. Paralysis of tongue
   - Kali.phos. 6x
   - Natrum sulph. 6x
   - Calc.sulph. 6x
5. Protrusion of tongue, difficult
   - Kali.phos. 6x
   - Natrum sulph. 6x
   - Calc.sulph. 6x
   - Silicea 6x
6. Soreness of tongue
   - Natrum sulph. 6x
   - Kali.sulph. 6x
   - Calc.sulph. 6x

TONICS

1. After acute sickness or fevers
   - Kali.phos. 6x
   - Natrum sulph. 6x
   - Calc.sulph. 6x
2. Boys -Tonic
   - Kali.phos. 6x
   - Natrum sulph. 6x
   - Calc.sulph. 6x
3. Children-Tonic
   - Ferrum phos 6x
   - Kali.sulph. 6x
   - Calc.sulph. 6x
4. Adults, men-Tonic
   - Natrum sulph. 6x
   - Kali.sulph. 6x
   - Calc.sulph. 6x
5. Girls - Tonic
   - Calc.phos. 6x
   - Kali.phos. 6x
   - Natrum mur. 6x

6. Adults, women - Tonic
Kali.sulph. 6x
Calc.sulph. 6x
Silicea 6x
7. Lactating mothers - Tonic
Kali.phos. 6x
Natrum sulph. 6x
Calc.sulph. 6x
8. Old age (men and women)-Tonic
Kali.phos. 6x
Natrum sulph. 6x
Calc.sulph. 6x

TONSILS

1. Hypertrophy, induration
Kali.sulph. 6x
Calc.sulph. 6x
Silicea 6x
2. Inflammation (Tonsillitis)
a. Acute tonsillitis
Kali.sulph. 6x
Calc.sulph. 6x
Silicea 6x
b. Acute, follicular tonsillitis
Kali.phos. 6x
Kali.sulph. 6x
Calc.sulph. 6x
c. Acute tonsillitis - pain radiating to ears
Kali.phos. 6x
Natrum sulph. 6x
Kali sulph. 6x
d. Chronic tonsillitis
Ferrum phos 6x
Natrum sulph. 6x
Kali.sulph. 6x

TOOTH ABSCESS

Nat.sulph. 6x
Kali.mur. 6x
Calc.sulph. 6x

TOOTHACHE
1. General formula
   - Kali.sulph. 6x
   - Calc.sulph. 6x
   - Calc.flor. 6x
2. Pain, after extraction of tooth
   - Kali.phos. 6x
   - Calc.sulph. 6x
   - Silicea 6x
3. Pregnancy, during
   - Mag.phos. 6x
   - Kali.sulph. 6x
   - Calc.sulph. 6x
4. Tobacco smoking, due to
   - Kali.phos. 6x
   - Natrum sulph. 6x
   - Calc.sulph. 6x
5. Throbbing toothache
   - Kali.sulph. 6x
   - Calc.sulph. 6x
   - Silicea 6x
6. With swelling about jaw, cheek (Gum-boil)
   - Ferrum phos 6x
   - Natrum sulph. 6x
   - Kali.sulph. 6x
   - Calc.sulph. 6x

(See Teeth also)

TORTICOLLIS (Wry neck-twisting of neck which tilts the head at an odd angle)
- Kali.phos. 6x
- Natrum sulph. 6x
- Calc.sulph. 6x

TOURETTE SYNDROME (Tics) (Sudden movements twitches, or sounds produced repeatedly. Repeated blinking)

Natrum sulph.	6x
Calc.sulph.	6x
Silicea	6x

TRACHOMA (See Eyes, Granular lids)

TRICHOPHYTOSIS (See Ringworm)

TRICHOTILLOMANIA (Compulsive hair pulling)

Natrum sulph.	6x
Kali.sulph.	6x
Calc.sulph.	6x

TRIGEMINAL NEURALGIA

Ferrum phos	6x
Natrum sulph.	6x
Calc.sulph.	6x

TRISMUS (Lockjaw) (Chewing muscles of jaw are contracted and inflamed and mouth can not be opened)

Kali.phos.	6x
Natrum sulph.	6x
Calc.sulph.	6x

TUBERCULOSIS
1. General formula

Natrum sulph.	6x
Kali sulph.	6x
Calc.sulph.	6x

2. Bones - tuberculosis

Kali.sulph.	6x
Calc.sulph.	6x
Silicea	6x

3. Intestinal tuberculosis

Calc.phos.	6x
Kali.phos.	6x
Natrum sulph.	6x

4. Pulmonary (lung) tuberculosis

Natrum sulph.	6x
Kali.mur.	6x
Calc.sulph.	6x

5. Extra-pulmonary (other organs) - tuberculosis
   - Natrum sulph. 6x
   - Kali.sulph. 6x
   - Calc.sulph. 6x

TUBERCULOSIS – (other diseases caused by tuberculosis)
1. Diarrhoea - due to tuberculosis
   - Natrum sulph. 6x
   - Kali.sulph. 6x
   - Calc.sulph. 6x
2. Digestive disorders - due to tuberculosis
   - Natrum sulph. 6x
   - Kali.sulph. 6x
   - Calc.sulph. 6x
3. Dyspnoea (breathlessness) - due to tuberculosis
   - Kali.phos. 6x
   - Natrum sulph. 6x
   - Calc.sulph. 6x
4. Emaciation, weight loss - due to tuberculosis
   - Kali.phos. 6x
   - Natrum sulph. 6x
   - Calc.sulph. 6x
5. Fever, due to tuberculosis
   - Kali.phos. 6x
   - Kali.sulph. 6x
   - Calc.sulph. 6x
6. Haemoptysis, due to tuberculosis
   - Kali.sulph. 6x
   - Calc.sulph. 6x
   - Silicea 6x
7. Haemoptysis, due to other causes
   - Kali.phos. 6x
   - Kali.sulph. 6x
   - Calc.sulph. 6x

TUMORS
1. Benign (non-cancerous) tumors
   - Kali.phos. 6x
   - Natrum sulph. 6x
   - Calc.sulph. 6x

2. Cancerous - tumors
- Kali.phos. 6x
- Natrum sulph. 6x
- Kali.sulph. 6x
- Calc.sulph. 6x

3. Cystic - tumors
- Kali.phos. 6x
- Natrum sulph. 6x
- Calc.sulph. 6x

4. Bone like protuberances - tumors
- Kali.phos. 6x
- Kali.sulph. 6x
- Calc.sulph. 6x

5. Fibroid, bleeding - tumors
- Kali.phos. 6x
- Natrum sulph. 6x
- Kali.sulph. 6x
- Calc.sulph. 6x

6. Lipoma (fatty tumors)
- Natrum sulph. 6x
- Kali.sulph. 6x
- Calc.sulph. 6x

7. Ployps - tumors
- Calc.phos. 6x
- Kali.phos. 6x
- Kali.mur. 6x

TYMPANIC MEMBRANE RUPTURE
- Natrum sulph. 6x
- Kali.sulph. 6x
- Calc.sulph. 6x

TYPHOID FEVER (Enteric fever)
- Kali.phos. 6x
- Natrum sulph. 6x
- Kali.sulph. 6x
- Calc.sulph. 6x

TYPHOID FEVER - CONCOMITANTS
1. Delerium, confusion, dizziness
   - Kali.phos. 6x
   - Natrum sulph. 6x
   - Calc.sulph. 6x
2. Diarrhoea - with typhoid fever
   - Kali.phos. 6x
   - Natrum sulph. 6x
   - Calc.sulph. 6x
3. Ecchymoses - with typhoid fever
   - Kali.phos. 6x
   - Natrum sulph. 6x
   - Calc.sulph. 6x
4. Epistaxis - with typhoid fever
   - Natrum sulph. 6x
   - Kali.sulph. 6x
   - Calc.sulph. 6x
5. Headache - with typhoid fever
   - Kali.phos. 6x
   - Natrum mur. 6x
   - Kali sulph. 6x
6. Haemorrhage - with typhoid fever
   - Kali.phos. 6x
   - Natrum sulph. 6x
   - Kali sulph. 6x
7. Pneumonia, bronchial symptoms, cough, with typhoid
   - Kali.sulph. 6x
   - Calc.sulph. 6x
   - Silicea 6x

TYPHUS FEVER (A group of bacterial diseases, transmitted to humans through lice, chiggers and fleas)
   - Natrum sulph. 6x
   - Kali.sulph. 6x
   - Calc.sulph. 6x

U

ULCERATIVE COLITIS (Chronic inflammation of colon and rectum with ulcers in their mucous membranes)

Natrum sulph.	6x
Kali.sulph.	6x
Calc.sulph.	6x

ULCERS - SKIN

1. General formula-ulcers in skin

Kali.phos.	6x
Natrum sulph.	6x
Calc.sulph.	6x

2. Bleeding, easiy, when touched

Natrum mur.	6x
Kali.mur.	6x
Calc.sulph.	6x

3. Deep ulers - skin

Kali.phos.	6x
Natrum sulph.	6x
Calc.sulph.	6x

4. Eroding ulcer, of face

Kali.phos.	6x
Natrum sulph.	6x
Calc.sulph.	6x

5. Fistulous ulcers- in skin

Kali.sulph.	6x
Calc.sulph.	6x
Silicea	6x

6. Scrofulous ulcers-in skin

Kali.phos.	6x
Kali.sulph.	6x
Calc.sulph.	6x

7. Sensitive ulcer - on skin

Kali.phos.	6x
Natrum sulph.	6x
Calc.sulph.	6x

8. Traumatic ulcers (due to injury)
Kali.phos.	6x
Natrum sulph.	6x
Calc.sulph.	6x

9. Varicose ulcers (due to varicose veins)
Kali.phos.	6x
Natrum sulph.	6x
Kali.sulph.	6x
Calc.sulph.	6x

ULCER

1. With base, blue or black
Natrum sulph.	6x
Calc.sulph.	6x
Silicea	6x

2. With discharge, fetid, purulent
Kali.sulph.	6x
Calc.sulph.	6x
Silicea	6x

3. With, edges, deep punched out
Kali.sulph.	6x
Calc.sulph.	6x
Silicea	6x

4. With, edges, irregular
Kali.sulph.	6x
Calc.sulph.	6x
Calc.flor.	6x

UMBILICUS
1. Bleeding from, in newborn

    Natrum sulph. 6x
    Kali.sulph. 6x
    Calc.sulph. 6x

2. Pain and inflammation (children and adults)

    Kali.sulph. 6x
    Calc.sulph. 6x
    Silicea 6x

UNCONSCIOUSNESS (See Syncope, Faintig)
UREA - RAISED

    Kali.mur. 6x
    Kali.sulph. 6x
    Calc.sulph. 6x

UREMIA

    Natrum sulph. 6x
    Kali.sulph. 6x
    Calc.sulph. 6x

UREMIA-Symtoms and complications
1. Appetite, loss of - in uremia

    Kali.phos. 6x
    Natrum sulph. 6x
    Kali.sulph. 6x
    Calc.sulph. 6x

2. Anemia - in uremia

    Kali.sulph. 6x
    Calc.sulph. 6x
    Silicea 6x

3. Coma - in uremia

    Kali.phos. 6x
    Natrum mur. 6x
    Kali.sulph. 6x
    Calc.sulph. 6x
    Silicea 6x

4. Convulsions - in uremia

    Kali.phos. 6x
    Kali.mur. 6x
    Calc.sulph. 6x

5. Itching, pruritus, skin - in uremia
   - Natrum sulph. 6x
   - Kali.sulph. 6x
   - Calc.sulph. 6x
6. Mental changes: anxiety and others - in uremia
   - Kali.phos. 6x
   - Natrum sulph. 6x
   - Calc.sulph. 6x
7. Metallic taste - in uremia
   - Natrum sulph. 6x
   - Kali.sulph. 6x
   - Calc.sulph. 6x
8. Muscle cramps - in uremia
   - Kali.sulph. 6x
   - Calc.sulph. 6x
   - Silicea 6x
9. Nausea - due to uremia
   - Kali.sulph. 6x
   - Calc.sulph. 6x
   - Silicea 6x
10. Smell in breath of uremia patient (ammonia smell)
    - Kali.phos. 6x
    - Natrum sulph. 6x
    - Calc.sulph. 6x
11. Urine formation stopped, by kidneys - in uremia
    - Natrum mur. 6x
    - Calc.sulph. 6x
    - Silicea 6x
12. Vomiting - in uremia
    - Kali.sulph. 6x
    - Calc.sulph. 6x
    - Silicea 6x
13. Weakness and easy fatigue - in uremia
    - Kali.phos. 6x
    - Kali.mur. 6x
    - Calc.sulph. 6x

14. Weight loss - in uremia
    - Kali.sulph. 6x
    - Calc.sulph. 6x
    - Silicea 6x

URETHRA
1. Bleeding from urethra
    - Natrum sulph. 6x
    - Kali.sulph. 6x
    - Calc.sulph. 6x
2. Burning in urethra
    - Natrum sulph. 6x
    - Kali.sulph. 6x
    - Calc.sulph. 6x
3. Burning, when not urinating
    - Kali.sulph. 6x
    - Calc.sulph. 6x
    - Silicea 6x
4. Discharge of transparent mucus secretion
    - Natrum sulph. 6x
    - Kali.sulph. 6x
    - Calc.sulph. 6x
5. Discharge of pus, from urethra
    - Kali.sulph. 6x
    - Calc.sulph. 6x
    - Silicea 6x
6. Inflammation of urethra (urethritis) (See Gonorrhoea)
    - Natrum sulph. 6x
    - Kali.sulph. 6x
    - Calc.sulph. 6x
7. Itching in urethra
    - Natrum sulph. 6x
    - Kali.sulph. 6x
    - Calc.sulph. 6x
8. Pain in urethra
    - Kali.sulph. 6x
    - Calc.sulph. 6x
    - Silicea 6x

9. Stricture in urethra
   - Natrum sulph. 6x
   - Kali.sulph. 6x
   - Calc.sulph. 6x

10. Urethral Fever (due to catheter)
    - Kali.sulph. 6x
    - Calc.sulph. 6x
    - Silicea 6x

URIC ACID, RAISED (Hyperuricemia)
- Natrum sulph. 6x
- Kali.sulph. 6x
- Calc.sulph. 6x

URAINARY BLADDER - DISEASES

1. Burning-in urinary bladder
   - Mag.phos. 6x
   - Nat.phos. 6x
   - Natrum sulph. 6x

2. Dribbling of urine
   - Kali.phos. 6x
   - Natrum sulph. 6x
   - Calc.sulph. 6x

3. Inflammation of urinary bladder (Cystitis)
   - Calc.sulph. 6x
   - Kali.sulph. 6x
   - Silicea 6x

4. Not emptied completely - bladder
   - Natrum sulph. 6x
   - Kali.sulph. 6x
   - Calc.sulph. 6x

5. Pain in bladder
   - Kali.sulph. 6x
   - Calc.sulph. 6x
   - Silicea 6x

URINARY FLOW - DESIRE
1. Constant desire - to urinate
    - Calc.sulph. 6x
    - Calc.flor. 6x
    - Silicea 6x
2. Frequent desire - to pass urine
    - Natrum mur. 6x
    - Kali.mur. 6x
    - Calc.sulph. 6x
3. Frequent desire, at night - to urinate
    - Natrum sulph. 6x
    - Kali.sulph. 6x
    - Calc.sulph. 6x
4. Irresistable, sudden desire - to pass urine
    - Kali.phos. 6x
    - Kali.sulph. 6x
    - Calc.sulph. 6x

URINARY FLOW
1. Intermittent urine flow (stops and starts repeatedly)
    - Kali.sulph. 6x
    - Calc.sulph. 6x
    - Silicea 6x
2. Involuntary urine flow (enuresis)
    - Kali.phos. 6x
    - Natrum sulph. 6x
    - Calc.sulph. 6x
3. Involuntary urine flow, at night (nocturnal enuresis)
    - Kali.phos. 6x
    - Natrum sulph. 6x
    - Silicea 6x
4. When coughing, sneezing (stress incontinence)
    - Natrum sulph. 6x
    - Kali.mur. 6x
    - Calc.sulph. 6x

URINARY TRACT INFECTION
- Natrum sulph. 6x
- Kali.sulph. 6x
- Calc.sulph. 6x

URINE, RETENTION OF (Ischiuria)
1. General formula
   - Kali.phos. 6x
   - Natrum sulph. 6x
   - Kali.sulph. 6x
   - Calc.sulph. 6x
2. From inflammation of bladder - (urine stopped)
   - Calc.sulph. 6x
   - Kali.sulph. 6x
   - Silicea 6x
3. From paralysis of bladder - (urine stopped)
   - Silicea 6x
   - Calc.sulph. 6x
   - Kali sulph. 6x
4. From delivery (after Labor) - (urine stopped)
   - Kali.sulph. 6x
   - Calc.sulph. 6x
   - Calc.flor. 6x
   - Silicea 6x
5. From prostatic hypertrophy - (urine stopped)
   - Calc.sulph. 6x
   - Silicea 6x
   - Kali.sulph. 6x
6. From surgical operation - (urine stopped)
   - Kali.sulph. 6x
   - Calc.sulph. 6x
   - Silicea 6x

URINE
1. Scanty flow (less in amount), due to decreased glomerular filtration rate (GFR)
   - Kali.sulph. 6x
   - Calc.sulph. 6x
   - Silicea 6x
2. Drop by drop - urine
   - Natrum sulph. 6x
   - Kali.sulph. 6x
   - Calc.sulph. 6x

URINE, SUPPRESSION (Anuria - no urine formation)
Natrum mur. 6x
Calc.sulph. 6x
Silicea 6x

URINATION
1. Complaints before passing the urine
   Kali.phos. 6x
   Natrum sulph. 6x
   Calc.sulph. 6x
2. Complaints during passing the urine
   Natrum sulph. 6x
   Kali.sulph. 6x
   Calc.sulph. 6x
3. Complaints after passing the urine
   Ferrum phos 6x
   Natrum sulph. 6x
   Calc.sulph. 6x

URINE
1. Sensation as if urine remained behind in bladder
   Kali.phos. 6x
   Natrum sulph. 6x
   Calc.sulph. 6x
2. Tenesmus, urging, straining, (while passing urine)
   Kali sulph. 6x
   Calc.sulph. 6x
   Silicea 6x

URINE - TYPES
1. Acidic urine
   Kali.phos. 6x
   Natrum sulph. 6x
   Calc.sulph. 6x
2. Alkaline urine
   Natrum sulph. 6x
   Calc.sulph. 6x
   Silicea 6x
3. Albuminuric - urine (See Abuminuria)
4. Bloody, hematuuria (See Hamaturia)

5. Burning, hot - urine
   - Ferrum phos   6x
   - Kali sulph.   6x
   - Calc.sulph.   6x
6. Oily, pellicle, on surface of urine
   - Kali.phos.   6x
   - Natrum sulph.   6x
   - Calc.sulph.   6x
7. Milky urine
   - Natrum sulph.   6x
   - Kali.sulph.   6x
   - Calc.sulph.   6x
8. Red, dark urine
   - Kali.phos.   6x
   - Kali.sulph.   6x
   - Calc.sulph.   6x

URINE - ODOR

1. Offensive, bad smell, in urine
   - Kali.sulph.   6x
   - Calc.sulph.   6x
   - Silicea   6x
2. Pungent, ammoniacal, urine
   - Kali.phos.   6x
   - Natrum sulph.   6x
   - Calc.sulph.   6x
3. Sharp, strong smell in urine
   - Natrum sulph.   6x
   - Kali.sulph.   6x
   - Calc.sulph.   6x
4. Sour smell in urine
   - Kali.sulph.   6x
   - Calc.sulph.   6x
   - Silicea   6x

URINE, SEDIMENT-TYPES

1. Bile sediment
   - Natrum sulph. 6x
   - Calc.sulph. 6x
   - Silicea 6x
2. Casts (cylindrical, tubular, granular casts)
   - Kali.phos. 6x
   - Natrum sulph. 6x
   - Calc.sulph. 6x
3. Cells and debris, in urine
   - Natrum sulph. 6x
   - Calc.sulph. 6x
   - Silicea 6x
4. Chlorides, diminished - in urine
   - Kali.phos. 6x
   - Natrum sulph. 6x
   - Calc.sulph. 6x
5. Grayish white, granular - sediments in urine
   - Natrum sulph. 6x
   - Kali.sulph. 6x
   - Calc.sulph. 6x
6. Hematuria (blood in urine)
   - Natrum sulph. 6x
   - Kali.sulph. 6x
   - Calc.sulph. 6x
7. Hematuria, gross, visible with naked eye
   - Kali.mur. 6x
   - Kali.sulph. 6x
   - Calc.sulph. 6x
8. Hematuria, microscopic
   - Calc.phos. 6x
   - Kali.mur. 6x
   - Calc.sulph. 6x

9. Hemoglobinuria (Hemoglobin in urine)
   - Natrum mur. 6x
   - Kali.mur. 6x
   - Calc.sulph. 6x

10. Oxalates, excessive - in urine
    - Natrum sulph. 6x
    - Calc.sulph. 6x
    - Silicea 6x

11. Pus in urine (Pyuria)
    - Kali.phos. 6x
    - Natrum sulph. 6x
    - Calc.sulph. 6x

URTICARIA (Hives)

1. General formula
   - Natrum mur. 6x
   - Kali.mur. 6x
   - Calc.sulph. 6x
2. From emotional problems - urticaria
   - Kali.phos. 6x
   - Natrum mur. 6x
   - Calc.sulph. 6x
3. From gastric derangements - urticaria
   - Natrum sulph. 6x
   - Kali.sulph. 6x
   - Calc.sulph. 6x
4. From menstrual disorders - urticaria
   - Kali.phos. 6x
   - Natrum sulph. 6x
   - Calc.sulph. 6x
5. Seuqellae or bad effects - from suppressed hives
   - Kali.phos. 6x
   - Natrum sulph. 6x
   - Calc.sulph. 6x

UTERUS

1. Atony, weakness of uterus
   - Kali.phos. 6x
   - Natrum sulph. 6x
   - Calc.sulph. 6x
2. Cervix of uterus - inflammation
   - Calc.phos. 6x
   - Kali.sulph. 6x
   - Calc.sulph. 6x
3. Cervix of uterus - tumor
   - Kali.phos. 6x
   - Natrum sulph. 6x
   - Calc.sulph. 6x
4. Cervix of uterus - ulcer, erosion
   - Natrum sulph. 6x
   - Kali.sulph. 6x
   - Calc.sulph. 6x
5. Fibroids-uterus
   - Kali.sulph. 6x
   - Calc.sulph. 6x
   - Calc.flor. 6x
6. Displacements, prolapse of uterus
   - Kali.phos. 6x
   - Natrum sulph. 6x
   - Calc.sulph. 6x
7. Inflammation of uterus (Metritis)
   - Kali.sulph. 6x
   - Calc.sulph. 6x
   - Silicea 6x

8. Pain, bruised broken feeling in uterus
   Natrum sulph.   6x
   Calc.sulph.   6x
   Silicea   6x
9. Pain, pressing down, as if uterus would come out
   Natrum sulph.   6x
   Kali.sulph.   6x
   Calc.sulph.   6x

V

VACCINATION, injection, or by mouth, ill-effects of

Kali.sulph.	6x
Kali.mur.	6x
Silicea	6x

VAGINA DISEASES OF
1. Aphthous, erosions - in vagina

Natrum sulph.	6x
Kali.sulph.	6x
Calc.sulph.	6x

2. Fungal infection (candidisis) (See Candidiasis)
3. Inflammation of vagina (Vaginitis)
   a. Acute vaginitis

Kali.sulph.	6x
Calc.sulph.	6x
Silicea	6x

   b. Chronic vaginitis

Kali.phos.	6x
Natrum sulph.	6x
Calc.sulph.	6x

4. Pain in vagina (Vulvodynia)

Natrum sulph.	6x
Kali.sulph.	6x
Calc.sulph.	6x

5. Prolapse of vagina

Calc.phos.	6x
Kali.phos.	6x
Natrum sulph.	6x
Kali.mur.	6x

VALVULAR DISEASES, OF HEART
1. General formula

Natrum mur.	6x
Kali.sulph.	6x
Calc.sulph.	6x

2. Mitral stenosis
    - Kali.phos. 6x
    - Natrum sulph. 6x
    - Calc.sulph. 6x
3. Aortic regurgitationand mitral regurgitation
    - Nat.sulph. 6x
    - Kali.mur. 6x
    - Calc.flor. 6x

VARICOCELE (Enlargement of veins in the scrotum)
- Natrum sulph. 6x
- Kali.sulph. 6x
- Calc.sulph. 6x

VARICOSE ULCERS (See Ulcer)
VEINS - DISEASES OF
1. Engorged, distended veins (Varicose veins)
    - Calc.sulph. 6x
    - Calc.flor. 6x
    - Silicea 6x
2. Inflamed veins (Phlebitis)
    - Natrum sulph. 6x
    - Kali.sulph. 6x
    - Calc.sulph. 6x
3. Inflammation of veins - chronic
    - Natrum mur. 6x
    - Kali.mur. 6x
    - Calc.sulph. 6x
4. Varicose veins - legs
    - Natrum sulph. 6x
    - Kali.sulph. 6x
    - Calc.sulph. 6x

VERTEBRA
1. Caries, Collapse, Necrosis - vertebra
 - Natrum sulph. 6x
 - Calc.sulph. 6x
 - Silicea 6x
2. Degenerative disc disorders, the space reduced
 - Natrum sulph. 6x
 - Kali.sulph. 6x
 - Calc.sulph. 6x
3. Bulging of vertebral disc
 - Calc.sulph. 6x
 - Natrum sulph. 6x
 - Calc.flor. 6x

VERTIGO – TYPES
1. General formula
 - a. Kali.phos. 6x
   - Calc.phos. 6x
   - Ferrum phos. 6x
 - b. Kali.mur. 6x
   - Natrum sulph. 6x
   - Silicea 6x
2. Decreased blood circulation of brain - due to
 - Kali.phos. 6x
 - Natrum sulph. 6x
 - Calc.sulph. 6x
3. Gastro-enteric derangements - due to
 - Natrum sulph. 6x
 - Calc.sulph. 6x
 - Silicea 6x
4. Old age (senile vertigo) - due to
 - Calc.sulph. 6x
 - Natrum sulph. 6x
 - Kali sulph. 6x
5. When traveling in car, vertigo
 - Kali.phos. 6x
 - Natrum sulph. 6x
 - Silicea 6x

6. When walking, vertigo

      Natrum sulph. 6x
      Kali.sulph. 6x
      Calc.sulph. 6x

VIRAL INFECTIONS - ALL TYPES AND SYMPTOMS
(See flu, influenza, coryza, cough, fever, pharyngitis, bronchitis, viral diseases, severe acute respiratory syndrome, asphyxia, cyanosis, avian influenza, septicemia, bird flu, cyanosis, multiple organ dysfunction syndrome, bronchospam, cough, pneumonia, swine flu, coma, blood clotting, clotting of blood and oxygen-low saturation, Yellow fever, Dengue fever, Ebola virus, MERS, Zika virus and other relevant symptoms).

VISION - DISORDERS
1. Amaurosis (Partial or total blindness)
      Kali.phos. 6x
      Natrum mur. 6x
      Natrum sulph. 6x
2. Amblyopia (Blurred, weak vision)
      Natrum mur. 6x
      Natrum sulph. 6x
      Calc.sulph. 6x
3. Blurred vision
      Kali.phos. 6x
      Calc.sulph. 6x
      Calc.flor. 6x
4. Blindness-Causes
 a. Blindness, due to headache
      Kali.phos. 6x
      Natrum mur. 6x
      Calc.flor. 6x
 b. Blindness, due to head injury
      Kali.sulph. 6x
      Calc.sulph. 6x
      Calc.flor. 6x

   c. Blindness, due to retinal detachment
- Kali.phos. 6x
- Kali.mur. 6x
- Calc.flor. 6x

   d. Sudden blindness, due to retrobulbar neuritis, or optic neuritis
- Kali.mur. 6x
- Kali.sulph. 6x
- Calc.sulph. 6x

5. Color-blindness
- Ferrum phos 6x
- Kali.mur. 6x
- Calc.sulph. 6x

6. Day-blindness
- Ferrum phos 6x
- Kali.sulph. 6x
- Calc.sulph. 6x

7. Diplopia (double vision)
- Natrum mur. 6x
- Kali.mur. 6x
- Kali sulph. 6x

8. Night-blindness
- Kali.sulph. 6x
- Calc.sulph. 6x
- Silicea 6x

9. Optical illusions

   a. Flashes, flames, stars
- Kali.phos. 6x
- Natrum mur. 6x
- Kali sulph. 6x

   b. Halo around light
- Natrum mur. 6x
- Kali.mur. 6x
- Calc.sulph. 6x

c. Spots, floaters (muscae volitantes)
        Kali.sulph. 6x
        Calc.sulph. 6x
        Calc.flor. 6x

10. Short-sightedness (Hypermetropia - weak distant vision)
        Ferrum phos 6x
        Natrum mur. 6x
        Kali.mur. 6x

11. Far-sightedness (myopia - weak near vision)
        Kali.phos. 6x
        Natrum mur. 6x
        Calc.sulph. 6x

VITILIGO (White patches on skin due to lack of melanin)
        Ferrum phos. 6x
        Natrum sulph. 6x
        Kali sulph. 6x

VITREOUS OPACITIES
        Natrum sulph. 6x
        Calc.sulph. 6x
        Silicea 6x

VOCAL CORDS
1. Inflammation of vocal cords
        Calc.sulph. 6x
        Natrum sulph. 6x
        Silicea 6x

2. Nodules on vocal cords
        Natrum sulph. 6x
        Kali.sulph. 6x
        Calc.sulph. 6x

3. Paralysis of vocal cords
        Kali.phos. 6x
        Natrum sulph. 6x
        Calc.sulph. 6x

VOICE – LOSS OF
1. Infection of larynx

    Ferrum phos 6x
    Natrum sulph. 6x
    Calc.sulph. 6x

2. Due to hemiplegia

    Kali.phos. 6x
    Natrum sulph. 6x
    Calc.sulph. 6x

3. Hysterical, loss of voice

    Kali.phos. 6x
    Natrum mur. 6x
    Kali sulph. 6x

VOMITING
1. Drinks of any kind

    Kali.phos. 6x
    Natrum sulph. 6x
    Calc.sulph. 6x

2. Eating, drinking

    Kali.phos. 6x
    Natrum sulph. 6x
    Silicea 6x

3. Gastric irritation

    Kali.phos. 6x
    Natrum sulph. 6x
    Calc.sulph. 6x

4. Milk

    Natrum sulph. 6x
    Kali.sulph. 6x
    Calc.sulph. 6x

5. Pregnancy

    Natrum sulph. 6x
    Kali.sulph. 6x
    Calc.flor. 6x

VOMITING - TYPES
1. Acid, sour vomiting

    Natrum sulph. 6x
    Calc.sulph. 6x
    Silicea 6x

2. Bilious (green or yellow) vomiting
   - Natrum sulph. 6x
   - Kali.sulph. 6x
   - Silicea 6x
3. Bloody vomiting
   - Natrum sulph. 6x
   - Calc.sulph. 6x
   - Kali sulph. 6x
4. With collapse, fainting, weakness - vomiting
   - Kali.phos. 6x
   - Kali.sulph. 6x
   - Silicea 6x
5. With fruitless retching - vomiting
   - Kali.sulph. 6x
   - Calc.sulph. 6x
   - Silicea 6x

VULVA - LABIA

1. Inflammation (Vulvo-vaginitis)
   - Calc.phos. 6x
   - Calc.sulph. 6x
   - Silicea 6x
2. Itching or pain-vulva
   - Natrum sulph. 6x
   - Kali.sulph. 6x
   - Calc.sulph. 6x

W

WARMTH (See Aggravation and Amelioration)
1. Aggravated of complaints, by warmth or heat
   - Kali.phos. 6x
   - Natrum sulph. 6x
   - Calc.sulph. 6x
2. Amelioration of complaints, by warmth or heat
   - Natrum mur. 6x
   - Kali.mur. 6x
   - Calc.flor. 6x

WARTS (Verruca)
1. Bleed easily, large warts
   - Calc.sulph. 6x
   - Natrum sulph. 6x
   - Kali.phos. 6x
2. Condylomata, fig-warts
   - Natrum sulph. 6x
   - Kali.sulph. 6x
   - Calc.sulph. 6x
3. Situated on body, anywhere - warts
   - Kali.phos. 6x
   - Natrum sulph. 6x
   - Calc.sulph. 6x
4. On face, hands - warts
   - Calc.sulph. 6x
   - Natrum sulph. 6x
   - Kali.phos. 6x
5. On genito-anal region - warts
   - Calc.sulph. 6x
   - Natrum sulph. 6x
   - Kali sulph. 6x

WEAKNESS, EXHAUSTION (See Neurasthenia also)
1. General formula
   - Kali.phos. 6x
   - Natrum mur. 6x
   - Calc.sulph. 6x

2. Abortion, repeated, due to
   - Kali.mur. 6x
   - Kali.sulph. 6x
   - Calc.sulph. 6x
3. From acute diseases, mental strain - weakness
   - Kali.phos. 6x
   - Natrum mur. 6x
   - Kali.sulph. 6x
4. From excessive use of drugs - weakness
   - Natrum sulph. 6x
   - Kali.sulph. 6x
   - Calc.flor. 6x
5. From excesses, vital drains - weakness
   - Natrum mur. 6x
   - Natrum sulph. 6x
   - Kali.mur. 6x
6. Grief - weakness, from
   - Kali.phos. 6x
   - Natrum mur. 6x
   - Kali.mur. 6x
7. From heat of Summer, heat exhaustion or heat stroke
   - Natrum mur. 6x
   - Kali.sulph. 6x
   - Calc.sulph. 6x
8. From jaundice - weakness
   - Natrum sulph. 6x
   - Kali.mur. 6x
   - Kali.sulph. 6x
9. Mental strain causes - weakness
   - Natrum mur. 6x
   - Natrum sulph. 6x
   - Kali.mur. 6x

10. In old age - weakness
> Calc.phos. 6x
> Kali.phos. 6x
> Natrum mur. 6x

11. Sedentary life style - weakness
> Natrum mur. 6x
> Natrum sulph. 6x
> Kali.mur. 6x

12. Sex, excessive indulgence, causes weakness
> Natrum mur. 6x
> Kali.mur. 6x
> Calc.sulph. 6x

13. Women, due to repeated pregnancies - weakness
> Kali.phos. 6x
> Natrum sulph. 6x
> Calc.sulph. 6x

14. Worse from exertion, walking - weakness
> Natrum mur. 6x
> Natrum sulph. 6x
> Calc.sulph. 6x

Worse, worn out due to hard mental and physical work, or luxury
> Kali.mur. 6x
> Kali.sulph. 6x
> Calc.sulph. 6x

WHEAT INTOLERANCE
> Ferrum phos 6x
> Natrum mur. 6x
> Calc.sulph. 6x

WHIP LASH INJURY (Neck injury due to back and forth jerk to head)
> Kali.sulph. 6x
> Calc.sulph. 6x
> Silicea 6x

WHITLOW (Herpetic Viral infection of thumb or fingers)
> Kali.sulph. 6x
> Calc.sulph. 6x
> Silicea 6x

WHOOPING COUGH
                Kali.phos.   6x
                Natrum sulph.   6x
                Calc.sulph.   6x

WILSON DISEASE (Deposition of copper in liver, brain and other organs)
                Natrum sulph.   6x
                Kali.sulph.   6x
                Calc.sulph.   6x

WISDOM TOOTH ERUPTION-difficult with pain and swelling
                Ferrum phos   6x
                Kali.sulph.   6x
                Calc.flor.   6x

WOLF-PARKINSON-WHITE SYNDROME (Abnormality in electrical system of heart leading to fast rate of heart)
                Natrum sulph.   6x
                Kali.sulph.   6x
                Calc.sulph.   6x

WORM FEVER
                Calc.sulph.   6x
                Natrum sulph.   6x
                Kali sulph.   6x

WORMS, intestinal
    1. Ancylostoma duodenale (hookworm)
                Calc.sulph.   6x
                Kali.sulph.   6x
                Natrum sulph.   6x
    2. Ascaris lumbricoides (roud worm)
                Natrum sulph.   6x
                Kali.sulph.   6x
                Calc.sulph.   6x
    3. Entrobius vermicularis (pin worm)
                Calc.sulph.   6x
                Calc.flor.   6x
                Silicea   6x

4. Oxyuris vermicularis
Kali.sulph.	6x
Natrum sulph.	6x
Calc.sulph.	6x

5. Taenia Saginata (Beef tapeworm)
Kali.phos.	6x
Natrum sulph.	6x
Calc.sulph.	6x

6. Taenia solium (Pork tapeworm)
Ferrum phos	6x
Natrum sulph.	6x
Calc.sulph.	6x

WORRIES - ill-ffects of
Kali.phos.	6x
Natrum mur.	6x
Silicea	6x

WOUNDS

1. General formula
Ferrum phs.	6x
Kali.mur.	6x
Calc.phos.	6x

2. Bleed profusely
Natrum sulph.	6x
Kali.sulph.	6x
Calc.sulph.	6x

3. Bullet, from
Kali.phos.	6x
Natrum sulph.	6x
Calc.sulph.	6x

4. Incised; surgical operation
Calc.sulph.	6x
Kali.sulph.	6x
Natrum sulph.	6x

5. With gangrenous tendency
Calc.sulph.	6x
Kali.sulph.	6x
Natrum sulph.	6x

WRIST DISEASES
1. Ganglion (cyst) on back of wrist
   - Calc.phos. 6x
   - Kali.phos. 6x
   - Natrum mur. 6x
2. Pain in wrist
   - Natrum sulph. 6x
   - Kali.sulph. 6x
   - Calc.sulph. 6x
3. Cramps, painful spasm (Writer's cramps)
   - Mag.phos. 6x
   - Natrum sulph. 6x
   - Kali.phos. 6x
4. Rheumatic, joint inflammation and pain in wrist
   - Calc.sulph. 6x
   - Natrum sulph. 6x
   - Kali.phos. 6x
5. Paralysis of wrist (wrist drop)
   - Calc.phos. 6x
   - Kali.phos. 6x
   - Calc.sulph. 6x

WRITER'S CRAMPS (See Wrist)

XERODERMA PIGMENTOSUM (XP)-(Severe sensitivity to sun light)
- Kali.phos. 6x
- Natrum mur. 6x
- Kali.mur. 6x

YAWNING, EXCESSIVE
- Kali.sulph. 6x
- Calc.sulph. 6x
- Silicea 6x

YEAST INFECTIONS
1. Candidiasis
   - Calc.sulph. 6x
   - Natrum sulph. 6x
   - Silicea 6x

2. Thrush

    Calc.sulph. 6x
    Natrum sulph. 6x
    Kali.phos. 6x

YELLOW FEVER

    Calc.sulph. 6x
    Kali.sulph. 6x
    Silicea 6x

ZOLLINGER ELLISON SYNDROME (Excess gastric acid)

    Calc.sulph. 6x
    Natrum sulph. 6x
    Kali sulph. 6x

www.ingramcontent.com/pod-product-compliance
Lightning Source LLC
Chambersburg PA
CBHW071909210526
45479CB00002B/350

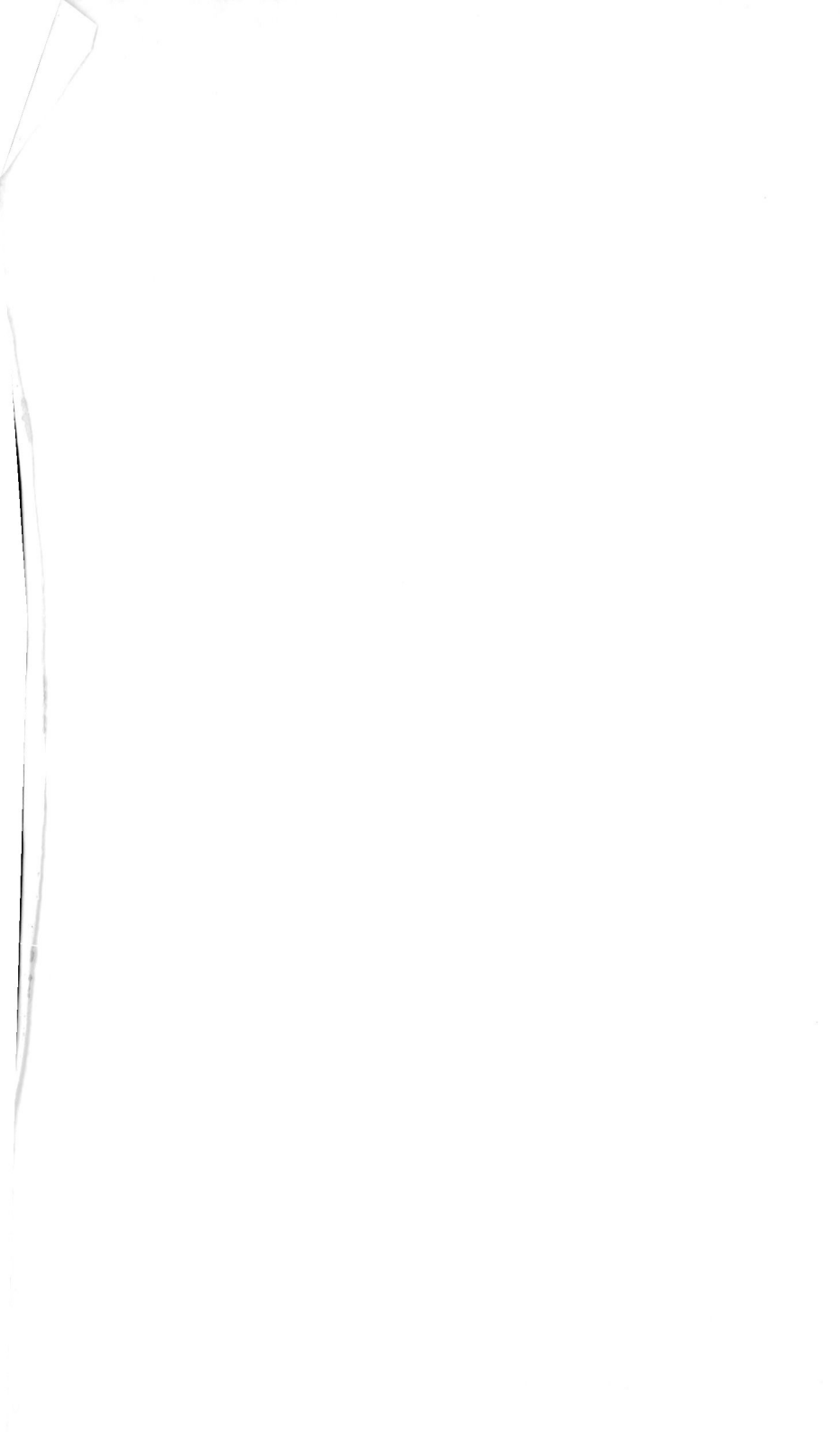